STRENGTH
TRAINING FOR
TRIATHLETES

2nd EDITION

STRENGTH TRAINING FOR TRIATHLETES

THE COMPLETE PROGRAM TO BUILD TRIATHLON POWER, SPEED, AND MUSCULAR ENDURANCE

PATRICK HAGERMAN, EdD

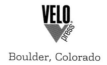

Boulder, Colorado

Before embarking on any strenuous exercise program, including the training described in this book, everyone, particularly anyone with a known heart or blood-pressure problem, should be examined by a physician.

Ironman® is a registered trademark of World Triathlon Corporation.

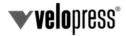

3002 Sterling Circle, Suite 100
Boulder, Colorado 80301-2338 USA
(303) 440-0601 · Fax (303) 444-6788 · E-mail velopress@competitorgroup.com

Distributed in the United States and Canada by Ingram Publisher Services

A Cataloging-in-Publication record for this book is available from the Library of Congress.
ISBN 978-1-937715-31-1

For information on purchasing VeloPress books,
please call (800) 811-4210, ext. 2138, or visit www.velopress.com.

This paper meets the requirements of ANSI/NISO Z39.48-1992 (Permanence of Paper).

Cover design by Andy Omel
Cover photograph by Nils Nilsen
Interior design by Vicki Hopewell
Interior photographs by Jeff Nelson
Gym location courtesy of Anytime Fitness, Boulder, Colorado
Composition by Jessica Xavier

Text set in Hoboken High and Dispatch

15   16   17 / 10   9   8   7   6   5   4   3   2   1

CONTENTS

Preface

Ever since the early 1960s, sport scientists and coaches have been looking for ways to make athletes bigger, faster, and stronger. While the science behind strength training is continually evolving, the principles of strength training haven't changed wildly over the years. The best way to become stronger is really quite simple: Lift heavy stuff. However, when you are using strength training to prepare for a specific sport, it becomes more complex. Every sport places different physical demands on the body, so there isn't one clear method that delivers the results every athlete is looking for. It's particularly challenging to design a strength training program for a triathlete, who is training for three sports.

Pick up any fitness magazine and there will be plenty of training trends, new exercises, and fad programs touted as the latest and greatest way to improve your speed, strength, or endurance. You can even find a fair number of strength training programs that are "designed" for triathletes. Unfortunately, many of the programs you will come across online, in magazines, or in talking with other athletes are not a good fit for your goals, your body, and your training schedule. To truly produce results, a strength training program must be specific to swim, bike, run while taking into account your individual strengths and weaknesses.

What sets this book apart is the fact that it doesn't play into the trends or fads, and it doesn't give you a one-size-fits-all program. This book will help you design a strength training program that does exactly what you need it to do—whether that be improving your speed, addressing a muscular imbalance, or overcoming a weak area. The science behind this program design has been proven over and over, and it is based on what a triathlete's body needs.

This second edition takes the groundwork that was laid in the first edition and builds upon it with the latest research in sport science. You will find more triathlon-specific exercises to keep training interesting, more sample programs to map the countless approaches you can take to strength training, and more options for at-home and travel workouts. Every exercise includes photographs to better illustrate good technique and execution. At the back of the book you'll find some useful charts to help with selecting exercises that focus on particular muscle groups and calculating the right weight to use for different goals over the course of your training.

As an athlete, you are always looking for a competitive edge, a training program that will put you on the podium or simply make you faster than you are now. This new edition of *Strength Training for Triathletes* can do just that.

PART I

STRENGTH TRAINING PROGRAM COMPONENTS

CHAPTER 1

Strength Training Versus Endurance Training

Triathlon is an endurance sport, plain and simple. So why should you consider strength training a necessary part of a triathlon workout? The short answer is that strength training makes muscles stronger, and stronger muscles can perform longer at higher intensities before they fatigue. To fully understand what is happening during strength training and endurance training you must break down and examine the subtle differences and similarities between the two. This book takes the long route because when you understand how the body works, it's much easier to plan training programs that work to your advantage.

Making the Case for Strength Training

If you ask any triathlete what endurance training is, the most common answer has something to do with swimming, cycling, or running. Technically, endurance training is any type of exercise that is rhythmical, maintains an increased heart rate and oxygen consumption, and uses large muscle groups to propel the body. It is also referred to as aerobic training because the body relies on a continuous, increased supply of oxygen during the energy-making processes at the cellular level. This supply of oxygen comes from increased respiration, usually the result of taking deeper breaths and breathing more frequently. In addition to increased respiration, the heart must pump more blood to the muscles to deliver the oxygen. So there is an increase in heart rate and respiration that is maintained throughout exercise: That's endurance training.

▬▬ STRENGTH TRAINING can be any type of training that increases the endurance, size, power, or strength of the specific muscles being used, regardless of what type of exercise is being done.

Ask the same triathlete what strength training is, and the answer usually involves some sort of weight lifting. In the most literal sense, strength training can be any type of training that increases the endurance, size, power, or strength of the specific muscles being used, regardless of what type of exercise is being done or whether someone is actually "pumping iron." Strength training is done in short bouts, with rest periods interspersed throughout the workout; is not rhythmical; and involves many different muscle groups, some large and some small. Strength training is considered anaerobic, or without oxygen. Even though you are breathing and your body is delivering oxygen to the muscles, the processes that provide energy for strength training do not rely on oxygen as the aerobic processes do.

Another difference between strength and endurance training is that strength training does not improve the cardiovascular system to any great extent. Each exercise requires a short burst of effort that doesn't require large increases in blood flow from the heart. During endurance training, as the heart rate rises, the heart is doing more work, so the heart muscle must be able to keep up the pace. To do this, the cardiac muscle tissue gets stronger, and the heart becomes more efficient at pumping blood. During strength training, significant, sustained increases in heart rate don't occur, and increases in oxygen delivery to the muscles are not needed, so the heart doesn't have to become stronger or more efficient.

The energy systems involved in endurance and strength training also differ in what they use as fuel. Along with delivering oxygen to muscles, the blood carries glucose (blood sugar) to the working muscles, where it is used as energy, stored as glycogen, or stored as fat. During endurance training, a large and steady supply of energy is required over a long period of time, so glucose is broken down to provide that energy and to allow the processes that burn fat stores to continue. You do not store enough glycogen in your muscles to sustain exercise for very long, so more glucose must be delivered by the blood to keep you moving. During strength training, the body must supply energy quickly but not in large amounts, so you use stored adenosine triphosphate and phosphocreatine (ATP-PC), along with the stored glycogen in your muscles. These energy systems provide a quick burst of energy, which is fine because a set of a strength training exercise doesn't take very long, and then you get to rest. Very little glucose or fat stores are used during strength training.

Anatomically, there is a great difference between strength and endurance training, but there are also some areas where the two overlap. Think about how often you lift weights during a triathlon. Other than lifting a cup of water to your mouth, taking your bike off the rack, and maybe picking yourself up off the ground, you don't lift that much—or do you? When you stop thinking of weight as a piece of iron attached to a barbell or machine, you realize that your body is a weight that you must lift and move all the time—and your muscles do the work. When you run, your legs have to push and hold up your entire body weight. When you swim, your arms help pull your body forward against the resistance of the water; and when you ride, your arms support your upper body as your legs push against the forces of the bike and pedals to propel you forward. In fact, we are continually lifting weight during endurance training and racing. It may not seem like much weight, but over the course of an endurance training session your muscles become fatigued from all that lifting, and your heart gets tired from all that pumping.

If strength training makes our muscles stronger, then it makes sense that swimming, cycling, and running make our muscles stronger, because we are working with the weight of our bodies. The weight is just a mass of muscle and bones rather than iron plates. You have probably experienced your muscles becoming stronger as a result of your swimming, cycling, or running program. If so, then congratulations—you have been doing a form of strength training all along.

You may be tempted to stop here, deciding that endurance training provides all the strength training you care to (or need to) do. After all, if your body weight is the only thing you are lifting during a triathlon, why would you need a training program that uses free weights or machines? But if what you have been doing were good enough to bring you the performances you want, you probably wouldn't be reading this book.

The problem with solely relying on your body weight to increase strength during endurance training is that your weight cannot provide adequate stimulus to bring about significant adaptation—your body is already used to it. To produce improvement in any type of training program, there has to be an overload, and the only way to provide it is to first make your body carry that weight in longer training sessions. But longer training sessions will not improve your performance and speed for shorter distances, so you have to add external weight in a manner the body is not accustomed to; that's how you create the correct stimulus.

▬ To produce improvement in any type of training program, there has to be an OVERLOAD.

Here's an analogy that may better explain this concept. Say you have a really cool muscle car, but it came with a tiny four-cylinder engine, so it doesn't go very fast or have much power. You take it to the repair shop, where the basic engine is replaced with a big, strong V8 engine. Now you can speed along as fast as you like and have plenty of power to pass slower cars. Your body is just like the muscle car. If you keep the same body but change the engine that moves it, so that it's stronger and has more power, then your athletic performances will improve and you will be passing slower competitors. Strength training creates a more powerful engine than if you were to rely on endurance training alone.

Obviously the mechanics of a conventional strength training program using some form of free weights or machines are quite different from those of conventional endurance training used by triathletes (swimming, cycling, and running). However, the type of strength training you do should directly benefit your swimming, cycling, and running. This is called sport-specific strength training. It mimics the movements of the sport, uses the same muscles used in the sport, and is applied in such a way that the intensity promotes the sport. Strength training for triathletes isn't a matter of just going to the gym and using whatever machine you find there; it has to be done in a deliberate and efficient way for you to achieve the desired physiological outcomes.

A physiological outcome is the way the body changes—in this case, how your muscles adapt. Four possible physiological outcomes can be achieved through a strength training program:

Muscular endurance: the ability of a muscle to withstand repeated use over a period of time.

Muscular hypertrophy: an increase in muscle mass, or size.

Muscular power: the ability to move the body quickly through the use of very fast muscular contractions.

Muscular strength: the amount of weight that the muscles can move in a single effort.

It's very important to remember that strength training doesn't necessarily mean you will bulk up. Far too often I hear the excuse, "I don't want to lift weights because it will make my muscles too big." That's just a simplistic generalization of what happens during strength training. Increased size is only one possible outcome, and you don't have to train for hypertrophy if you don't need to. Each of these outcomes has a place in a triathlete's training program. How you achieve each one is covered in Chapter 2. The key is to achieve just the right amount of each outcome at just the right time.

How Strength Training for Triathletes Is Different

Strength training routines can be wildly different depending on the sport they are intended to complement and on an individual athlete's needs. What constitutes a successful sport-specific strength training program for one triathlete may not work as well for another triathlete. It all depends on your level of training, the length of the triathlon you are training for, and your individual needs. But one thing is universally true: Strength training for triathletes should be very different from programs used by bodybuilders, powerlifters, and the general public. Everyone has the same muscles and bones, but everyone uses them in completely different ways. Different training goals, or outcomes, are reached by using different combinations of exercises, sets, repetitions, rest periods, exercise order, weight, and progression plans.

SAID Principle

Specific Adaptations to Imposed Demands is the basis for sport-specific training. This means that your body will adapt in a very specific way based on the demands that you impose on it during training. For example, to make your arms stronger, you have to train your arms, not your legs; or in endurance terms, to become a better swimmer, you have to swim, not run.

For example, a bodybuilder is interested in one thing: size. In their case, the bigger the muscle, the better. Having large, bulging muscles is not what a triathlete wants, because body mass negatively affects endurance efficiency, and larger muscles add a lot of mass but not necessarily a lot of strength. The bigger your muscles are, or the more mass they have, the more strength it takes to move that mass, especially over a long distance. Mass also creates increased frontal resistance in the water and frontal air resistance on land.

However, the triathlete can benefit from larger muscles if that increased size is kept in check and is used properly. If you want to increase the performance of a muscle, sometimes you have to start by increasing its size. After all, you can't make a muscle stronger if you don't have enough muscle to begin with. Once the muscle size is where it needs to be, you can change the emphasis of your strength training to move toward your desired outcome. A muscle that is the right size can be made stronger and more powerful or be given more endurance. So don't immediately rule out using a strength training program that focuses on hypertrophy, because it may be exactly what you need. For example, most of us have a dominant side that includes an arm or leg that is larger and stronger than the other side. Most

▬ The triathlete can BENEFIT from larger muscles if that increased size is kept in check and is used properly.

right-handed people will have larger muscles in their right shoulder compared to their left. People who drive a lot have larger calf muscles in their right leg because of all the "reps" they do pushing the accelerator pedal. Sometimes we need to focus on hypertrophy to even out the body. Additionally, if you have ever suffered a serious injury that required rehabilitation, there is a good chance that one limb is larger than the other. This happens when rehab is focused on the injured limb and neglects the unaffected limb—allowing only one limb to get stronger or larger. On the other hand, long-term rehab, in which both limbs are used, allows the unaffected limb to get stronger or larger while the injured limb progresses more slowly. In each case you have a unilateral deficiency in both size and strength that could be fixed with focused strength training with hypertrophy as the goal.

Athletes who compete in powerlifting and weightlifting are not usually as big as bodybuilders; however, they are very strong for their size. In these sports, success depends on how much you can lift, not on how big you look. Powerlifters who compete in contests for bench press, squat, and deadlift, as well as weightlifters competing in the Olympic lifts—the snatch and the clean and jerk—are usually very strong for their size. (Some of the strongest lifters pound for pound are actually women.) But remember, these heavyweight sports have almost no endurance component, because a competitive lift consists of 1 rep that will last anywhere from 2 to 20 seconds. A triathlete needs compact, strong muscles but requires much more endurance from them.

General fitness programs are likewise not useful for triathletes, mainly because of their wide range of variety and their lack of sport-specific exercises. Training for general fitness is more about

> ### Endurance Efficiency
>
> Endurance efficiency is the amount of energy you use per pound of body weight during aerobic training. The goal for triathletes is to be very efficient by having lean, strong muscles, not large, weak muscles.

working all the different parts of the body in a manner designed to work as many muscles at one time as possible, often using machines that are designed to make the exercise comfortable rather than to mimic a sport's movement. So although most of the exercise programs you find in popular magazines will improve your fitness, they won't do much to improve your triathlon performances. The key is to choose exercises that mimic the sport of triathlon and put them together in a way that works for you.

How Strength Training Leads to Better Performance

You will more than likely boost your race results if you incorporate strength training into your triathlon training, because stronger muscles deliver increased power, speed, lean mass, and muscular endurance. Your race focus, experience level, and current body composition will inform how these benefits contribute to your performance gains.

Muscular Power

The first benefit of strength training is muscular power, or the ability to produce force quickly. In a triathlon this is useful during a short sprint to pass a competitor, uphill cycling, and transitioning into and out of the water. A powerful muscle is able to call upon its anaerobic

◼︎ When you have more muscle to rely on, it takes LONGER to wear it out.

energy stores to support quick movement. Strength training increases muscular power in two ways: (1) The more muscle you have, the less effort it takes to produce a given amount of power (remember the muscle car analogy), and (2) strength training teaches your muscles to reproduce energy quickly so they can better recover from short bouts of high-intensity movement. Energy production and recovery happen deep down in the muscle fibers, where glycogen, enzymes that increase the speed of muscular contraction, and creatine and phosphocreatine (energy substrates) are all increased because of strength training.

Speed

Second, you can increase your speed through strength training, regardless of what race distance you compete in. This is the result of the selective recruitment of fast-twitch muscle fibers during strength training. During endurance training you mainly use your slow-twitch fibers, which are designed for low power output and long durations. During strength training you have to call upon the fast-twitch muscle fibers for their high power and force output. The downside to fast-twitch fibers is that they fatigue quickly—usually in less than five minutes. When you put out a sudden burst of speed in training or racing, you know that you cannot sustain it for very long before slowing back down to your regular pace. Strength training builds up the ability of the fast-twitch muscle fibers to activate and provide that burst of speed. You will still have to slow back down, but you can obtain a higher-intensity burst of speed (meaning faster) and recover from it faster, which means you can do it again when you need to.

Lean Mass

The third performance benefit of strength training comes from an indirect effect: a reduction in body fat because of an increase in lean mass. Decreasing one's body fat is typically equated with losing fat, but the equation has two sides—you can also increase lean tissue. Endurance training burns a lot of fat, but it doesn't build much lean tissue. Strength training is all about increasing lean tissue. Again, we are not talking about bulking up your muscles, but about making the muscles you have more dense. Increasing muscle density decreases your fat-to-lean ratio, which ultimately improves performance. Fat doesn't assist in movement—it's just along for the ride, which increases the demand on the muscle to move it along. More lean tissue means more muscle to produce movement, which is exactly what you want, because muscle essentially carries itself.

Muscular Endurance

Finally, increasing muscular strength increases muscular endurance. When you have more muscle to rely on, it takes longer to wear it out. If you find that you sometimes reach muscular fatigue before you reach cardiovascular fatigue, then you should increase your muscular strength so that you have more in reserve. Endurance training decreases cardiovascular fatigue; strength training increases muscular endurance, which in turn decreases muscular fatigue.

Considerations for Your Strength Training Plan

Training for Different Distances

Strength training programs for triathletes often employ similar exercises, but differ depending on the race distance you are training for. Performing well in a shorter sprint race calls for more speed and power than muscular endurance, whereas an Ironman®-distance event requires less speed and power and more muscular endurance. In between those you have the Olympic and half-Iron distances, which require a combination of speed and endurance. So each race distance necessitates a strength training program with different outcomes. The balance of each outcome with the training distance is probably the most important aspect of program design. Just as you wouldn't train like a bodybuilder and expect to perform well in a triathlon, a sprint-distance triathlete can't approach strength training in the same way as a triathlete who competes in Iron-distance events. The distance you strive for will affect the reps, sets, and weights you use (more on this in Chapter 2), as well as how often you can strength train in conjunction with your endurance training schedule. It all has to come together in just the right way for it to work. After an explanation of the specific components, later chapters provide more detailed information on putting together a program for each race distance.

Time Investment

If you have been a triathlete for some time, you know how many hours you need to put into your endurance training. At times it seems as though you're doing endless laps in the pool, thousands of mind-numbing pedal strokes, and long miles on the road. You may be thinking that you don't have time for strength training on top of that—there are only so many hours in a day, after all. Fortunately, strength training doesn't take very much time. In the beginning, if you can spare 30 minutes a day, three days a week, the results will make you want to do more. It's even possible to cut back on your endurance training to make room for strength training and end up with better endurance training sessions. How much time you want to invest is going to depend on your particular goals, but most strength training programs can be completed in a 30- to 45-minute workout if it is designed efficiently.

If you can spend 90 minutes a week increasing your body's ability to perform during all those other hours you train, won't it be worth it? Of course it will! Once you find the right combination of muscle density and efficiency, your leg turnover will become faster, your strokes more powerful, and your spinning quicker—all without a mindful increase in effort. That's the beauty of strength training: Not only do you feel stronger, but everything else improves as a result. And this happens very quickly. Your body will begin responding to a strength training program within the first couple of weeks, though you might not see anything different in the mirror right away because initially the changes will be happening on the inside.

■■■ **Once you find the RIGHT COMBINATION of muscle density and efficiency, your leg turnover will become faster, your strokes more powerful, and your spinning quicker—all without a mindful increase in effort.**

Fitting strength training into your busy life and training schedule can still be a challenge. While the *when* of strength training is one of those questions that science has not equivocally answered, you'll find out soon enough that if you strength train immediately before you do any endurance training, your muscles will be fatigued and your endurance training will suffer. Likewise, if you do your endurance training before you hit the weights, you'll find that you can't lift as much or with as much power. Fatigue is always going to be an issue. The solution is to split up your training sessions so they are at different times on the same day or on different days. This will be covered more in Chapter 2.

It is also possible to do too much strength training. The additional strain that strength training adds to your entire program can be too much if you don't ease into it and back off on your endurance training at the same time. Overtraining will set back your performance, extend the time it takes you to recover from injuries, and just plain slow you down. Nothing is worse than a muscle that won't heal because you pushed it too far. A proper strength training program must be put together with your entire training regimen in mind and without pushing your body too far. This book provides some guidelines to get you started in the right direction, but ultimately you need to listen to how your body responds and let it guide you toward the proper balance of strength and endurance training for you.

Intensity

Probably the most important component of your strength training program is the intensity, which is a combination of the weights you use, how much you rest between sets, and the length of a workout. To properly produce the efficiency you want, and to push the muscular endurance levels upward, the intensity has to be set so that you are constantly moving from one exercise to another, with enough rest between each set of an exercise to allow for some energy recuperation but not so much that you cool down before you start up again. The best way to do this is to group exercises together in repeating series called circuits. This is an advanced version of the circuit training programs that were popular during the 1980s but with more scientific rationale to make it effective.

Intensity is not just about how much weight you can lift. In fact, in many exercises the weight is just your body weight or a few extra pounds. How much weight you can move isn't the key to intensity; it's putting the right amount of resistance in the right place during the right movement. It all has to fit in with triathlon movements and

▰▰ INTENSITY changes during a triathlon, and it changes during a strength training session.

the muscles used in some specific way. Intensity changes during a triathlon, and it changes during a strength training session. As you learn the components of a good program and see how to put together an individualized program, you will learn how intensity can be manipulated to your benefit.

The Principle of Specificity at Work

Specificity is one of the most important concepts behind strength training for sports. As mentioned previously, sport strength training has to be designed to mimic the sport you are training for. The movements you produce during the swim, bike, and run can be mimicked in a weight room with a little creativity. Unfortunately, equipment manufacturers haven't produced a lot of triathlon-specific exercise machines, so many of the exercises in this book require some imagination, but they simulate the bigger movements involved in our sport. For example, a squat will definitely make your legs stronger, but when in a triathlon are you pushing off with both feet at the same time? Never! However, during cycling you extend the hip, knee, and ankle of one leg at a time, over and over. So all you have to do is develop an exercise that allows you to mimic this one-leg squat to create a sport-specific exercise for cycling. Keep this in mind as you flip through the book and try the exercises in Part III; they may still look unfamiliar, but you'll know why they work.

At the same time, an exercise that is not exactly sport specific can have a positive benefit for your sport. For example, football players spend a lot of time working on their bench press strength. If you think about a football game, if a player is lying on their back and pushing up, they are probably trying to get another player off of them—meaning the play is over. So the bench press isn't exactly a sport-specific exercise for football. Or is it? If you can picture the same bench press position, but standing, you can see how a football player who is standing up and pushing against another player is very sport specific. What does this have to do with triathlon? The point is that some exercises have a carryover effect that has little to do with the position you are in during the exercise. As mentioned earlier, a one-leg squat simulates the movement you use in cycling. However, if doing a one-leg squat is too difficult, then a two-leg squat is your solution. You will still get a strength benefit, and you will work both legs at the same time. It's not exactly a sport-specific movement, but it will improve your strength for cycling and maybe you will eventually be able to successfully complete the more sport-specific movement.

CHAPTER 2

By the Numbers: Reps, Sets, Weight, and Rest

Having established the merits of a strength training program, the next step is building your program based on sound scientific evidence. There are many strength training programs available, but unfortunately many of them just don't deliver the goods. A solid training program should be based on scientific evidence rather than on what the guy is doing on the treadmill next to you. The same goes for copying the training program of a successful athlete. Just because a training program produced results for another person doesn't mean it will do the same for you. How much your body changes with any training program will be determined by your genes. However, if you are using the most scientifically sound program available, one developed for your goals and strengths, you can take full advantage of what your parents gave you. This chapter is all about numbers—and in strength training, there are lots of numbers. Choosing the correct number of repetitions per set, the right number of sets, and the perfect amount of weight for each exercise, as well as resting just enough, is the way to get the results you want.

Different Reps for Different Goals

The number of reps you complete in each set of an exercise greatly influences the result of that exercise. As discussed in Chapter 1, the four main physiological results that can be achieved with strength training are muscular endurance, hypertrophy, power, and strength. This list shows the corresponding number of reps per set to achieve each goal:

Muscular Endurance	12–20 reps/set
Hypertrophy	6–12 reps/set
Power or Strength	1–6 reps/set

There is some overlap in the number of reps from one goal to the next. There are two reasons for this: First, when you train for one goal, you automatically receive a small amount of the benefits of each of the others. For example, if your training goal is strength, you will also become slightly more powerful, increase muscle mass a little bit, and have more muscular endurance. However, you will see the most significant changes come as a result of your main goal. If you train for strength, you will become stronger than if you trained for muscular endurance. On the opposite end of this continuum, if you are training for muscular endurance, you will also become slightly stronger, gain a small amount of muscle mass, and increase power just a little. This is called the carryover effect, and Table 2.1 illustrates how it plays out in training.

The second reason for the overlap is that science has not yet determined the optimum number of reps for each goal. Since the first research on strength training was published 70 years ago, these numbers have become more precise, and in another 10 years they will likely change more. Over time, the picture becomes clearer.

The range of reps for each goal also gives you some room to work and progress, which Chapter 3 will explore in more detail. Having a

TABLE 2.1. **CARRYOVER EFFECT OF STRENGTH TRAINING**

REPS	≤2 3 4 5 6	7 8 9 10 11	12 13 14 15 16	17 18 19 ≥20
	Muscular Endurance	Muscular Endurance	**MUSCULAR ENDURANCE**	
	Hypertrophy	**HYPERTROPHY**	Hypertrophy	Hypertrophy
Training Goal	**POWER**	Power	Power	
	STRENGTH	Strength	Strength	

range of reps is always better than having a single, preset number; allowing for normal day-to-day variations in training. Some days you may be feeling great, so you'll do extra reps. Other days you might not be at the top of your game, so you'll do fewer reps. Your program can handle these fluctuations, and as long as you stay within the range of reps for your goal, you'll remain on track.

In popular magazines that publish training programs, 10 seems to be the magic number of reps. However, there are no magic numbers in exercise science. Training programs that use 10 reps per set are most likely to make muscles bigger because this number falls on the high side of the hypertrophy range. Because a triathlete should not continually focus strength training on building bigger muscles, you should disregard many of the training programs available to the general public.

Single Versus Multiple Sets

There is an ongoing argument over whether to use a single set for each exercise or multiple sets per exercise. This stems from the fact that if you are doing nothing, one set of each exercise will provide noticeable benefits. However, this argument doesn't apply to athletes, because they are already involved in an exercise program of some sort. For athletes, a single set has clearly been shown to be inferior to multiple sets, but the exact number of sets you need has not been defined. What scientific research has shown is that for each goal there is a range of sets that provides the most benefit:

Muscular Endurance	2–3 sets
Hypertrophy	3–5 sets
Power or Strength	3–6 sets

Again, there is an overlap. There are fewer sets to complete for muscular endurance compared to strength, power, and hypertrophy. To some extent, there is an inverse relationship between the number of reps for each goal and the number of sets you complete. To develop muscular endurance, you are doing the most reps but the smallest number of sets. To focus on power and strength, you are doing the fewest reps but the most sets. This is all a function of exercise volume, which is the total amount of weight you lift during an exercise or workout. It is calculated by multiplying sets times reps times weight. Setting weight aside, a balance is created by adjusting the levels of sets and reps. As one goes up, the other goes down. This helps to keep the volume of exercise you do fairly even over time and as you progress through goals.

Another reason that the number of sets goes down as the number of reps goes up is to prevent overuse injuries. Even with a relatively light weight, doing rep after rep will eventually wear on your joints. To prevent this, the number of sets is decreased. As the weight gets heavier and you do fewer reps, there is less chance of repetitive motion injury, but you will need to do more sets to give your body enough stimulus to improve.

Choosing the Right Weight

The question I am asked most often is, how much weight should I use? Unfortunately, this is the most difficult question to answer because everyone has different capabilities. It is impossible to tell exactly how much weight you should use on every exercise unless you are tested on every exercise. This is where you will have to do some work to set up your own program. Reps and sets are universal numbers; weight is not. However, the method for determining how much weight to use is the same for everyone. It involves testing to determine your estimated 1-rep max (1RM)—the maximum amount of weight you can lift one time with correct form. This testing requires trial and error, but the method is straightforward. Once you have your estimated 1-rep max, you can use a percentage of that (% 1RM) to set your training goal.

Researchers have been working on finding the most appropriate percentage of this 1-rep max for each training goal but have yet to discover the best number, so again we will work within these ranges of resistance:

Muscular Endurance	50–67% 1RM
Hypertrophy	65–85% 1RM
Power or Strength	80–100% 1RM

Again, there is some overlap, for the same reasons that reps overlap. The most important point is that the amount of weight you use increases as you move from muscular endurance to hypertrophy to power or strength. This fits perfectly into our understanding of muscular endurance, which is about lifting a lighter weight numerous times, versus strength, which is about lifting a heavier weight a few times.

The number of reps you complete in any given set is inversely proportional to the weight you use. Put simply, the more something weighs, the fewer times you can lift it; the lighter it is, the more times you can lift it. So depending on your goal, not only will your reps change, but so will the weight you'll be using. Table 2.2 lists approximately how much weight you can lift (as a percentage of your 1-rep max) for a given number of reps.

TABLE 2.2. DETERMINING WEIGHT BASED ON YOUR 1-REP MAX

% 1RM	100	95	93	90	87	85	83	80	77	75	70	67
REPS	1	2	3	4	5	6	7	8	9	10	11	12

Estimating Your 1-Rep Max

To make this book applicable to everyone, instead of using actual weights in our program designs, we use percentages of your 1-rep max to describe how much weight to use in any given exercise. This does not apply to exercises that only use your body weight for resistance, since you can't use just a percentage of your weight—it's all or nothing. With any exercise that uses external weight for added resistance (squats and biceps curls, for example), using a percentage of your 1-rep max allows you to put together a program based on your goals and then plug in the actual weights you will use on each exercise. It also allows you to swap exercises in and out of your program without changing the goal of the program—so long as you keep using the appropriate percentage.

To decide how much weight to use, you will need to find out what your 1-rep max is for each exercise. There are two ways to go about this: (1) Actually do a maximum lift test for every exercise, or (2) complete a submaximal lift for each exercise and estimate the 1-rep max from that. Doing a maximum lift test for each exercise can be very tiring, and if you aren't skilled in an exercise, it can cause

Guidelines for Submaximal Testing to Find 1-Rep Max

1 Find a weight with which you can complete between 3 and 10 reps and perform as many reps as possible.

2 If you reach 11 reps, rest awhile, increase the weight, and repeat the test.

3 If you can do 3 to 10 reps, multiply the weight you used by the rep factor corresponding to the number of reps you completed (see Table 2.3).

acute injury that will delay your training. Using a submaximal lift and calculating your 1-rep max from that gives you a very close estimate without as much effort and risk of injury. Table 2.2 provides approximate calculations to help you get close enough (usually within a few pounds) for your needs.

The couple of workouts you spend testing will be more than worth the effort later. For each exercise, find a weight that you can lift between 3 and 10 times. If you can do 11 reps, increase the weight and try it again after a short rest. It doesn't matter if you can only do 3 reps, 7 reps, or 10 reps—as long as the number is between 3 and 10 you can calculate your 1-rep max by multiplying the weight you use by the corresponding rep factor shown in Table 2.3. For example, let's

TABLE 2.3. ESTIMATING YOUR 1-REP MAX WITH A SUBMAXIMAL TEST

REPS COMPLETED	3	4	5	6	7	8	9	10
REP FACTOR	1.10	1.13	1.16	1.20	1.23	1.27	1.32	1.36

say you completed 8 reps of the front raise exercise with 20 pounds. You would then multiply 20 pounds by the corresponding rep factor shown in Table 2.3 for 8 reps (1.27) to get an estimated 1-rep max of 25.4 pounds (20 × 1.27). It is not uncommon to end up with an estimate that includes a decimal point; you will deal with that later.

The next step involves calculating the amount of weight you actually want to use. Continuing with the same example, if your estimated 1-rep max is 25.4 pounds, and you choose to start training for muscular endurance, you would multiply the estimated 1-rep max by 65 percent. In this case, 65 percent of 25.4 pounds is 16.51 pounds. Of course the weights you find in the gym are usually in increments of 2.5 or 5 pounds. So in this case you would round 16.51 down to 15 pounds. Always round down rather than up, because it's better to go with a lighter weight and add more later than to use too much and risk injury. Again, the method isn't perfect, but it will help you get started, and then you can make refinements as you go.

Repeat this procedure for all the other exercises in your program. This will take some time, and you may have to adjust the trial weight several times until you find the right weight, but don't rush it. It's better to take your time and get this right. Use Appendix C to log your 1-rep max for each exercise and calculate the weight for each training goal.

■■ **RETEST your 1-rep max about every three months and adjust the weights you are using to keep your program within the correct ranges for your goal.**

As you train, your body adapts and becomes stronger, which means your 1-rep max will go up. This occurs no matter what goal you are training for, but it will happen faster if you are training for strength. Retest your 1-rep max about every three months and adjust the weights you are using to keep your program within the correct ranges for your goal. Three-month intervals should be long enough to show sufficient improvement to make the time spent testing and recalculating worthwhile. Doing it more frequently would use up training time to make very small changes that wouldn't make much difference in the weights you use.

Effects of Your Body Weight

So what about all the exercises that don't obviously involve weight? Remember that your body weight *is* weight; it *is* resistance that your muscles are working against. When you do a body weight exercise, you have to lift your entire weight, or at least the weight of the part of your body that is moving. Because you can't lift a percentage of your body weight, you can't make pull-ups or push-ups any easier unless you lose weight or get stronger. Most body weight exercises are shuffled into the category of muscular endurance training (provided that you can complete at least 12 reps). It is possible to increase the resistance of body weight exercises by adding ankle or wrist weights or wearing a weighted vest. But this turns them into weighted exercises instead of body weight exercises. You don't have to calculate an estimated 1-rep max for these exercises, because the weight is still your body weight plus a small amount; just stick with the correct number of reps for your goal.

Getting Enough Rest

It has been said that rest is the most important part of any training program. The improvements we see don't come about during training; they happen during the rest or recovery period in between training. That's when your body responds to the training and adapts to it in preparation for the next session. That being said, most serious triathletes engage in

■ The improvements we see don't come about during training; they happen during the rest or RECOVERY period in between training.

endurance training almost every day. Fortunately the body responds very well to daily training, as long as you have built up to this point slowly and know exactly how hard you can push yourself. The key to recovering from endurance training lies in its relatively low intensity spread out over the training session. It's easy for the body to recover from exercise that uses large muscle groups and doesn't stress any one system too much.

Strength training is a little different, however. Instead of working large groups of muscles, you may be focusing on individual muscle areas, single joints, and heavier loads over a number of reps and sets. This requires a different approach to rest.

Rest Between Sets

Getting the proper amount of rest between each set is important when designing a strength workout. To allow the anaerobic energy systems to recover enough to complete the next set, you have to rest, but not too much. There are several methods for determining the proper amount of rest, most based on subjective feelings rather than science. Some people rest long enough between sets to allow their heart rate to return to resting, some people let their breathing return to normal, and others like to have a cup of coffee or a nap between sets. According to the research, the amount of rest should be based on how fast your anaerobic energy systems recover. Do not allow your body to fully recover; let it recover just enough, so that the next set will be slightly more fatiguing. Making your body work with an incomplete recovery forces it to adapt. If you wait until you are totally recovered, your body will not have to get any better because it will be allowed to work within its capabilities. In general, it takes about 7 minutes to replenish 90 percent of your ATP (adenosine triphosphate, the energy that the anaerobic systems produce). In 3 minutes only about 50 percent of your ATP has been restocked. The strength training programs you will be doing won't totally deplete your ATP, so you don't have to wait this long between sets. That would make for a really long workout!

The amount of rest between sets that you need depends on your goal. Here's the breakdown:

Muscular Endurance	<30 sec.
Hypertrophy	30–90 sec.
Power or Strength	1.5–3 min.

The amount of rest is directly linked to the amount of energy provided by the anaerobic energy systems and the intensity of the exercise. For muscular endurance training, very little rest is needed because the intensity is low (50–67% 1RM), and the goal is to keep your muscles working as much as possible. In hypertrophy training you need a little longer between sets because the intensity is higher (65–85% 1RM). Finally, in power or strength training the low number

ATP

Adenosine triphosphate is the form of energy that your body uses to produce muscular contractions. Every form of food you eat (carbohydrates, fat, and protein), and the substrates it is converted to in the body (glucose, glycogen), is eventually broken down to make ATP. This is the only source of energy your body can use for movement.

of reps and the higher intensity (80–100% 1RM) require the most rest between sets. To allow enough rest between each set but not make your workout too long, stack your exercises in a circuit so that you are actually completing a set of a different exercise, using different muscles, while you are resting from the previous set. So while one muscle is resting, you are working another. You may have to stack two to three exercises in a circuit to allow enough time between sets for power or strength training, and you may choose not to stack any for muscular endurance training. Table 2.4 reviews all of the component ranges for each training outcome.

Rest Between Workouts

Endurance training can take place every day, but you wouldn't do the same workout every day because of the risk of overuse injury. The same goes for strength training. You can strength train every day, but you have to do different workouts so that your muscles can recover. Because of the higher-intensity work that your muscles do during strength training, the rule is to let them rest 48 hours before working them again. If you want to add strength training into your daily schedule, you just have to split your workout so that some muscles get to rest while others are working. A common approach is to split your workouts into upper- and lower-body days or to split up the muscle groups so that you train complementary muscles together on different days (split program). For example, you could do a two-day split working chest, triceps, and shoulders on Day 1. On Day 2 you could do exercises focused on legs, biceps, and back. Alternately, the workout could be split over three days: on Day 1 work legs and shoulders, Day 2 biceps and back, Day 3 chest and triceps. (Appendix A allows you to quickly reference the muscle groups.)

Complete rest occurs in 48 hours, but after 96 hours you actually get too much rest. How is that possible? If you rest too long,

TABLE 2.4. GUIDELINES FOR SETS, REPS, WEIGHT, AND REST

GOAL	SETS	REPS	WEIGHT	REST
Muscular Endurance	2–3	12–20	50–67% IRM	<30 sec.
Hypertrophy	3–5	6–12	65–85% IRM	30–90 sec.
Power or Strength	3–6	1–6	80–100% IRM	1.5–3 min.

your body will decide that it doesn't need to maintain its new level of ability, so it will actually start to downgrade. This is the basic "use it or lose it" rule. Everything you do in training is designed to improve your body systems, but your body is inherently lazy and wants to maintain minimal homeostasis (the least amount of work it has to do). So after 96 hours without another workout stimulus to keep it going, your body starts to return to baseline.

To prevent this decline, establish a routine for strength training with no more than two days of rest between workouts. For example, if you want to use an entire-body workout, you need to do it at least every three days. If you split up your workout into smaller pieces, make sure that you work each muscle group again between 48 and 96 hours later. Chapter 7 explores some training programs that you can use as guidelines.

Combining Strength and Endurance Training

Probably the most difficult part of adding strength training to your typical triathlon training is finding the time to do both. A typical strength training program will take about 30 minutes to complete, so it doesn't sound like much, but that can be time out of your usual endurance

■■■ Over time, your body will ADAPT to the increased workload of strength training, and the amount of fatigue you experience will decrease.

training, so something has to give. A second challenge with adding strength training is making sure that it doesn't make you too tired to complete your usual endurance training. As mentioned earlier, doing a strength training workout immediately before or after endurance training is going to affect the rest of your training. Your muscles can only do so much work before they become fatigued. Again, rest is the key to making it all work.

If you are already doing endurance training every day of the week, the best way you can incorporate strength training is to divide up your training into two sessions, separated by at least four hours of rest. One option is to do strength training in the morning, then endurance training in the evening—or vice versa. Another option is to complete your regular strength training workout, then modify your endurance training that day. You can shorten the endurance portion while increasing the intensity, simply cut it short, or work opposing muscle groups. For example, if your strength training that day focuses on upper-body and core exercises, do your run or bike training that day too (using mainly lower-body muscles). Swim training can be combined with lower-body and core exercises. There will inevitably be some duplication of muscles used, but that can't be avoided. The key is to minimize this so that you do not overwork or injure any one muscle group.

Over time, your body will adapt to the increased workload of strength training, and the amount of fatigue you experience will decrease. Luckily, science has provided some good evidence of what will happen when we combine strength and endurance training— also called concurrent training. Thus far, the research has shown that the increases in cardiorespiratory endurance, as measured by your VO_2max, are not affected by concurrent training. On the opposite end of the spectrum, concurrent training does not allow you to reach your strength potential, but blunts the effects of strength training at some point, which is different for everyone. This doesn't mean that you won't get stronger; you will. It just means that you won't get as strong as if you were doing strength training by itself. For the tri-athlete, this is perfectly fine because the strength benefits you need in order to improve your triathlon performances are well within the adaptations you will find before you hit that strength ceiling.

CHAPTER 3

Progression Systems: How to Keep Moving Forward

No strength training program will be successful if there isn't a plan for changing it once the body has adapted. The same is true for endurance training. Rather than setting a goal and stopping once you've achieved it, you set a new goal. In strength training, the goals aren't as specific as increasing your swim splits by a certain amount of time or running a particular distance; they are about continuously improving rather than getting to a certain point. There are several different ways of progressing a strength training workout, and different systems will work for different people. Contrary to what you may read elsewhere, no one system is inherently better than another. This chapter discusses some of the more commonly used systems for athletes, each of which has its advantages and strengths. You need to find one that works with your overall training program, and you may find that changing it up every now and then helps keep you motivated.

Principle of Overload

Progression is about effecting change in a program. When considering how to make a strength training program more difficult, often the first thing that comes to mind is increasing the weight, but in fact overload comes in many forms. The principle of overload states that for adaptation to occur, the body must be subjected to a stimulus that is greater than what it is used to. This stimulus can be in the form of more weight, repetitions, or sets; additional exercises; or less rest between sets. As long as what you choose makes the workout a little harder, that's overload.

Without overload, all you have is maintenance. Because you are seeking to do more than maintain your performance level, overload has to happen. As soon as you have adapted to a new overload, it is time to add another one. The progression systems in this chapter outline specific ways to know when adaptation has taken place and it is time for a new stimulus.

When deciding which component to change to produce overload, look at how each small change affects the entire workout. Exercise volume, mentioned in the discussion of sets and reps in Chapter 2, is affected by each of the other components. To begin with, volume is a calculation that basically tells you how much total weight you lifted during a workout. The equation is sets × reps × weight. Rest time is not part of the calculation because it is the only variable that makes a workout more difficult when it is reduced rather than increased. If you leave everything else in the equation as is and reduce the amount of rest between sets, that creates an overload, even though exercise volume hasn't changed. In addition, you must calculate volume for each exercise and add the volumes together to get a total for each workout. If you are using the same sets, reps, and weight for several exercises, you can modify the calculation to sets × reps × weight × number of exercises.

The smallest change you can make to volume is to add 1 rep to an exercise. Although that tiny change is an overload because it's more than you are used to, it is often not a significant one. On the other hand, adding another set increases volume significantly because you are adding several reps. Adding another exercise changes volume even more because you are adding several new sets. The effect of changing the weight you use depends on how much weight is added.

One of the best ways to determine whether your workout is successful is to track your exercise volume over time. Keeping track of exercise volume is simple, but you have to pay attention to all the numbers and not mix them up. Remember, if you are using different weights on several different exercises, you have to calculate the volume for each of those exercises individually and add them all together at the end.

Principle of Overload

This principle states that the body will only adapt, improve, and change when it is subjected to a stimulus that is greater than what it is used to. A lack of overload results in maintenance, or even loss of fitness.

The 2-for-2 Rule

The simplest form of progression that an athlete can use is linear progression, based on the 2-for-2 Rule, which states that when you can complete 2 additional reps on the last set of an exercise for 2 consecutive workouts, it is time to progress by adding a new overload. This new overload can be in the form of more reps, another set, less rest between sets, or more weight. The 2-for-2 Rule requires you to use a set number of reps and sets for each workout (3 sets of 15, for example). It also requires you to push yourself on the last set, when you are the most fatigued.

The 2-for-2 Rule takes into account that most people have good and bad days, when their ability to work out is improved or hampered by outside forces (nutrition, sleep, emotions, stress, etc.). On those days when everything falls into place and you are having a great workout, those extra 2 reps may be easy, but on days when you are struggling to even get through the workout, 2 additional reps may be completely out of the question. The 2-for-2 Rule prevents premature overload by making sure that the first time you achieved an extra 2 reps on the last set wasn't just a fluke. By doing consecutive workout performances with the extra 2 reps, you can be sure that you are actually ready to move forward. This is a simple way to gauge readiness to overload or change the workout. The next workout should have a new overload to challenge your new capability. Table 3.1 provides an example of exercise progression using the 2-for-2 Rule.

TABLE 3.1. EXAMPLE OF THE 2-FOR-2 RULE OF PROGRESSION

Keagen's program is focused on muscular endurance. His sets and reps for the upright row exercise are shown below. He completed 3 sets of 15 reps, plus 2 extra reps in set 3 in consecutive workouts. He increased the load to 30 pounds for the next workout and was no longer able to do the additional reps in the third set.

WORKOUT 1			WORKOUT 2			WORKOUT 3		
SET	REPS	WEIGHT	SET	REPS	WEIGHT	SET	REPS	WEIGHT
1	15	25	1	15	25	1	15	30
2	15	25	2	15	25	2	15	30
3	15+2	25	3	15+2	25	3	15	30

The 2-for-2 Rule progression strategy is great for athletes who like a simple workout plan without a lot of complicated numbers. Having a specific number of sets and reps for each workout makes everything straightforward. It also requires you to be able to push yourself when you are the most tired, which is especially challenging at the end of a workout.

Circular Progression

Circular progression is a little more complicated than the 2-for-2 Rule because you will work within the ranges of reps for each goal, rather than using a set number of reps for each set (refer to Table 2.4, page 31, for these ranges). In circular progression you start by establishing your goal for a particular exercise. For example, if you are training for hypertrophy, you will use between 6 and 12 reps for each set. Instead of trying to finish a certain number within the range, you will always strive to reach the highest number of reps for that goal (in this case, 12). So during every set, your goal is to get 12 reps. When you achieve 12 reps, it's time to progress by inserting a new overload. The most common, and easiest, component to change in circular progression is the weight.

If you add more weight to produce overload, you will complete fewer reps. This is exactly what you want to happen. If you make just a small increase in weight, your reps should still be within the range for your goal. For example, increasing weight reduces your reps on the next set from 12 to 8. Now you have to keep working with that weight until you can complete a set of 12 again. Then it's time to increase the weight again. As its name implies, this system keeps going around: increasing reps, then weight, then reps again, then weight again, and so on (Figure 3.1).

An important point to remember when using circular progression is that for it to work correctly, you have to put forth your best

FIGURE 3.1. **EXAMPLE OF CIRCULAR PROGRESSION**

Keagen's program is focused on hypertrophy. These are his sets and reps for the runner's raise. He started out using 25 pounds, and as soon as he completed 12 reps, he increased the weight to 30 pounds for the next set.

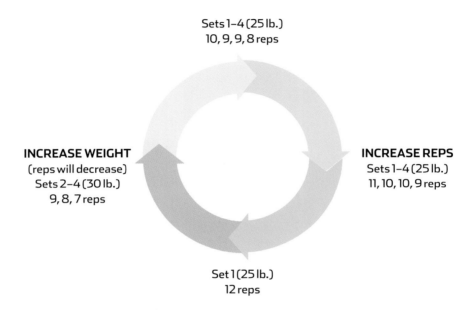

Sets 1–4 (25 lb.)
10, 9, 9, 8 reps

INCREASE WEIGHT
(reps will decrease)
Sets 2–4 (30 lb.)
9, 8, 7 reps

INCREASE REPS
Sets 1–4 (25 lb.)
11, 10, 10, 9 reps

Set 1 (25 lb.)
12 reps

effort on every set, especially the first. You should always complete the most reps on your first set, because you are the least fatigued when you start that set. If you do more reps on the second, third, or fourth set of an exercise, then you really weren't giving it your all at the beginning. When you do reach the maximum number of reps for your goal, the new overload must occur on the very next set. This differs from the 2-for-2 Rule, which allows for some variation in effort. Circular progression assumes that if you can do it once, you can do it again, so there is no waiting to make the overload adjustment.

The benefit of circular progression is that it makes ongoing adjustments based on your performance. You are not tied to a set number of reps but are allowed to push yourself constantly. In addition, because of the relationship between reps and weight, as long as you are training within the correct range of reps, you will also be using the correct percentage of your 1-rep max for your goal. You do not have to retest after you have made improvements; the exercise adjusts automatically with you. This style of progression requires a healthy amount of motivation from you, but if you give it your all, you will see improvements on a regular basis.

Periodization

Since the early 1990s, periodization of training programs has grown in popularity, starting with professional and Olympic athletes and working its way out to the general public. If planned and used correctly, periodization can offer some benefits that the 2-for-2 Rule and circular progression alone cannot. Periodization is so effective because it is built on the concept of sequenced potentiation, which is a method of building on previous goals or ability. For instance, you could train for more strength, or you could train first for hypertrophy, then for strength. The latter sequence takes the increased muscle size and builds strength from that, whereas the former just builds strength

Sequenced Potentiation

A training program that uses one goal to provide the foundation for the next goal and then builds on that foundation is using sequenced potentiation to generate greater results. It is the foundation, or stepwise approach, that allows the body to develop different physiological outcomes in a systematic way.

■ You can change the numbers to fit your training needs, schedule, and goals and always MAKE IMPROVEMENTS.

from the muscle you already have. If the goal is increased strength, periodization allows you to build up to a higher level of strength than a regular training program does.

Periodized programs are built one period at a time. The periods of training are grouped together to serve one overall goal, which could be muscular endurance, hypertrophy, strength, or power. Each period is called a cycle. The overall program is called the macrocycle, which has the overall goal. Within the macrocycle are two or more mesocycles, which divide the overall goal into smaller goals. Each of these smaller goals has a different physiological outcome, and each successive mesocycle builds on the results of the previous mesocycle. Finally, each mesocycle is divided into two or more microcycles, in which the actual component programming is done. Each microcycle builds on the previous microcycle, until the goal of the mesocycle is reached. Table 3.2 is a visual layout of a three-month periodization program with one-month mesocycles, each with two-week microcycles.

Periodization can be adapted to just about any length of time. You can use it between triathlons or to train for a single big one down the road. There are no rules about how long the macrocycle has to be, as long as you can fit at least two mesocycles within one macrocycle, and at least two microcycles within each mesocycle. A good rule of thumb is to keep microcycles at least one to two weeks long so that your body can have time to adapt toward one goal before you move on to the next.

Choosing the macrocycle and mesocycle lengths is simple. The real work is putting together your microcycles, because this is where

TABLE 3.2. **PERIODIZATION: 3-MONTH MACROCYCLE**

GOAL	WEEK	MICROCYCLE
Mesocycle 1	1–2	1-1
	3–4	1-2
Mesocycle 2	5–6	2-1
	7–8	2-2
Mesocycle 3	9–10	3-1
	11–12	3-2

the real progression takes place. The idea is to have each microcycle build on the next, with an overall scheme of increasing intensity and decreasing volume over the course of each entire mesocycle and macrocycle. For example, using Table 3.2 as a starting point, Table 3.3 fills in the goals and components. The first mesocycle has a goal of muscular endurance, the second hypertrophy, and the third strength. Within each mesocycle, the microcycles include each of the required sets, reps, and the percentage of the 1-rep max that correlates with the mesocycle goal. As the microcycles progress, we see an increase in intensity and a decrease in volume. Putting these numbers together is more an art than a science. As long as you stay within the ranges for each goal, and as long as the intensity rises and the volume decreases from microcycle to microcycle, you can't go wrong. There are numerous ways to use these guidelines to reach the same goal, which is another good thing about periodization. You can change the numbers to fit your training needs, schedule, and goals and always make improvements.

So far you have only covered the program components of sets, reps, and weight for your periodization program. You also have to

TABLE 3.3. **EXAMPLE OF PROGRESSION WITH PERIODIZATION PROGRAM**

Keagen's program is focused on building strength. He does a different circuit in eight exercises for each mesocycle (month). His workout volume is calculated by multiplying sets, reps, and weight for each exercise, and then taking the sum of all exercises. Volume decreases as load increases.

GOAL	%1RM	SETS	REPS	VOLUME
Muscular Endurance (Mesocycle 1)	60	3	20	3,600
	65	3	15	2,925
Hypertrophy (Mesocycle 2)	70	3	12	2,520
	75	4	8	2,400
Strength (Mesocycle 3)	85	4	6	2,040
	90	5	4	1,800

include the actual exercises you want to use. Again, there are no rules about which exercises to use or when to change them. In fact, you can use entirely different exercises for each microcycle—yet another way of introducing overload in this progression. When calculating your volume, the easiest way to incorporate the number of exercises you are using is to keep the number the same, for example, always using six exercises. But you can also start the program with basic exercises that you are good at and progress to more difficult exercises. This makes your body not only work harder as the program moves along, but learn new skills as well.

Tapering Strength Training Before a Race

As in any type of training program, in the days leading up to a competition you should reduce the amount and intensity of training to allow your body to fully recuperate prior to the event. With strength training, you should maintain intensity while decreasing frequency, then volume. Typically, tapering strength training 7 to 10 days before an event, with at least 3 full days of rest before the event, is suggested. Begin by decreasing the frequency of your training sessions, allowing more rest days between each one. If you are using a split program, switch to a full-body training program so that you can decrease the number of training days and not leave any muscle groups untrained. You may need to decrease the number of exercises you are using for each muscle group, so focus on those exercises that you feel will benefit you most.

Next, decrease exercise volume to a low level, but maintain the same intensity (amount of weight). Research has shown that you can maintain fitness levels for a short period of time if the intensity of training is maintained while the frequency and volume of training are decreased. This effect only lasts a short time before the body begins to lose fitness, so don't start tapering too early.

PART II

PROGRAM PREPARATION

CHAPTER 4

Strength Training Tools and Equipment

I n any health club, gym, or fitness center you will find a wide array of choices in exercise equipment. There are more than 50 manufacturers of gym equipment. In addition, late-night television commercials offer exercise techniques and special equipment that are supposed to provide results that no other products can. With all these choices, how do you know what equipment is useful and what just doesn't work?

When you're trying to build a strength training program that is specific for triathlons, not every exercise or piece of equipment will be right for you, even if it does work the right muscle. The equipment has to provide the correct stimulus to the appropriate muscle in the right direction. Unfortunately, not much equipment has been designed with triathletes in mind. Most equipment is built with ease of use and visual appeal in mind, and much of it doesn't do what it was intended to.

This chapter provides a foundation you can use to decide what equipment is right for you. Because more and newer designs are released every year, it is important that you be able to scrutinize equipment to get the best return for your money and effort.

Free Weights Versus Machines

There is a long-standing argument about whether free weights or exercise machines are better. Free weights have been around longer than machines. Ancient Greeks lifted different-sized rocks as exercise. There is a story about a man named Milo who supposedly lifted a bull calf every day of its life—effectively lifting more and more weight as the bull grew. In the early 1970s, Universal Equipment brought out a lineup of chrome-plated equipment that introduced exercise machines to the general public.

The question of whether free weights or machines are better is a trick question. No one piece or type of equipment is better than another; they are just different. What matters is exactly what you are trying to do and what equipment will provide that result.

A free weight is anything that provides resistance, is free to move in any direction, and is not attached to an immovable object or a base. Examples are weight plates, barbells, dumbbells, ankle weights, and even your body. A free weight doesn't have to be made of iron or steel, or even have a handle. A free weight can be just about anything you can pick up and move—a sack of groceries, your bike, or even your luggage.

A machine is a piece of equipment that only moves in one direction no matter how you push or pull on it. Machines are usually designed to do only one thing, such as knee extensions, so they cannot be used for other muscle groups, other joints, or any other motion. Therefore machines are relatively limited compared to free weights. Within the machine category, there are two distinct styles: plate-loaded and selectorized. Selectorized machines have a stack of plates for resistance. You choose the resistance by inserting a pin under the weight you want to use. Plate-loaded machines require you to add free-weight plates to the machine to increase resistance. They are sometimes marketed as a combination of free-weight and machine equipment, but the only free-weight component is picking up a plate and putting it on the machine, which is not part of the actual exercise.

A few factors really highlight the differences between machines and free weights. Machines provide a stable environment in which you only have to concentrate on moving the machine. They are safer than free weights because you can't drop them on your toes, they usually have a seat that provides support and extra leverage for pushing against, and they are easy to learn to use. Free weights require additional coordination and balance, which machines have built in. This extra work means that other muscles are being used to keep your posture and technique correct during the exercise. For example, if you use a biceps curl machine, the machine makes sure your arms are kept in the right place, you get to sit down so there is no upsetting your posture, and all you have to do is pull the weight up. On the other hand, using a free weight such as a barbell to do a biceps curl requires you to use your legs and back muscles to maintain a standing posture, especially as the weight is brought up, and there is a tendency to lean back to balance it. You have to maintain the correct arm position as well because there is no pad to rest against. Machines therefore have the advantage of making the exercise more focused (you don't have to do anything but pull on the weight), which can make them safer for beginners. On the other hand, because free-weight exercises require other muscles to provide support (your legs and back), they create a more realistic situation because your body is not supported at every angle. This is more difficult and requires more practice to maintain correct form.

Because a machine can only do one thing, sometimes there isn't one that works the movement you want to perform. However, you can accomplish just about every exercise imaginable with free weights if you use your imagination. Free weights don't take up much space and can be used for several exercises. You would have to have a different machine for every exercise in your program, so space becomes an issue really quickly for those considering a home gym.

Is there a machine that is better suited for the movement you want to perform, or is a free weight the better option? Depending on the exercise, how specific the movement is, and the amount of resistance you need to apply, the answer can go either way. Again, one is not better; they are just different. A combination of free-weight and machine exercises is used in later chapters, and each is chosen because of its practical application and benefits for the triathlete.

User-Defined Cables

Another type of equipment used often in this book is cables, technically called user-defined cables because the user decides how the equipment is used. For example, a low-pulley cable could be used for several different hip exercises, as well as for some upper-body exercises such as biceps curls. Cable equipment comes in several forms, from large, multistation pieces to single low- or high-pulley pieces to the newest styles that allow you to move the pulley anywhere from the floor to above your head with a simple adjustment.

User-defined cables are beneficial because they allow you to choose a movement that fits your body size and your particular movement patterns. A machine only moves in one direction, so you can't make adjustments to make it fit you. A cable moves where you tell it to move, so it always fits your body. A free weight should do the same thing, but a free weight only works when you are lifting the weight up, whereas a cable can be set so that you are pushing the handles (and therefore the resistance) directly out in front of you, or even down toward the ground. Because gravity only works in one direction with free weights, that limits their use for some movements.

Body Weight

Body weight as an important source of resistance during triathlon training has been discussed in Chapter 2. In fact, your body weight is the one type of resistance that you can't get rid of (unless you are training in outer space). Just the act of sitting up or standing is an exercise against gravity. When you are doing other strength training exercises, the weight of your body isn't usually figured into the amount of resistance, but it's always there. We don't count it because it is too difficult to measure. You can stand on a scale and see how much you weigh, but you never really lift your whole body weight. When doing a leg extension, you lift the weight you have selected, plus the weight of your leg from the knee down. How much more is that? It is not practical to weigh just part of your body, so we normally just accept that it's there and ignore it. This is fine, but be aware that it is part of the equation.

Resistance Tubing

Resistance tubing comes in several different forms. The most common and useful for your purposes is the style that has handles at both ends. Most tubing comes in lengths of about four feet, and there are several different thicknesses so that you can vary the resistance.

Resistance tubing uses potential energy to provide more resistance the more you stretch it. Potential energy describes the amount of energy an object has stored up as a result of its position. If you hold a dumbbell in the air, it has potential energy. As soon as you let go of it, it will fall to the floor and hit with a certain amount of force.

Unlike free weights or machines, which have a fixed amount of resistance, tubing's resistance becomes greater the farther you stretch it—to a point. For example, a 10-pound dumbbell is always going to weigh 10 pounds, but a piece of tubing may start out rela-

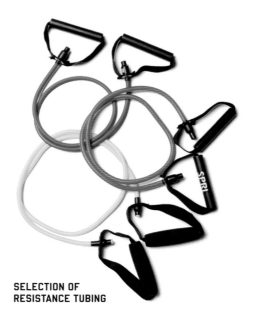

**SELECTION OF
RESISTANCE TUBING**

tively easy and become "heavier" as you stretch it. However, there is a point at which a piece of resistance tubing is stretched too much and the resistance drops. That is actually pretty hard to do, and would require it to be stretched to the point where it may break—think huge rubber band being snapped. If it does break, you can fix it by tying the two ends securely back together. The tubing will be a little shorter, but it will still work.

Choosing the correct tubing for a particular exercise involves trial and error. Tubing comes in a variety of resistances, ranging from easy to hard. Start with a lighter piece of tubing and move up to avoid injury. You can get several different types of tubing to give yourself a variety of resistance, or you can also double up and use two pieces of the same size tubing to double the resistance. When you make a piece of tubing shorter by choking up on the handles or wrapping it around a support pole a few times before starting your exercise, you effectively increase the resistance it will provide (but also the chance that it will stretch too far and break, so be careful).

Most exercises using resistance tubing require the tubing to be attached to an anchor so you can pull or push on the handles. If you have a machine or pole, you can simply wrap the tubing around it at various heights according to the exercise instructions. If you are exercising at home, a tubing anchor that is inserted through the opening between a door and the doorframe is the perfect solution. When the door is shut, the anchor provides a solid place to loop your tubing through, and the door will not be damaged. Never just shut the door on your tubing, thinking that the door will hold it in place; the tubing will tear.

Because resistance tubing can be anchored in any position, it's similar to a cable. The difference is in the resistance: The cable provides constant resistance, whereas the tubing has progressive resistance. If you find an exercise that requires cable equipment but do not have access to such equipment, you can substitute resistance tubing and perform the exercise exactly the same way.

Stability Balls

Stability balls are a great unstable platform for exercise and provide a support during exercises in which a regular exercise bench just can't do the job. They can take the place of any type of exercise bench or seat for most free weight and resistance tubing exercises and are an important part of some core exercises.

Stability balls come in several sizes. The right size for you depends on your height. When you sit on top of a stability ball, the tops of your thighs should be parallel to the floor. If your knees are higher than your hips, the ball is too short; if your knees are lower than your hips,

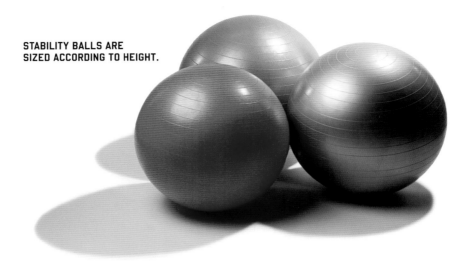

**STABILITY BALLS ARE
SIZED ACCORDING TO HEIGHT.**

the ball is too tall. Keep the ball properly inflated. It should flatten out somewhat when you sit or lie on it, but it should always be inflated enough that it rolls around under you. A ball that is too flat increases the stability of the platform, which defeats the purpose altogether.

Medicine Balls

Medicine balls are an old-fashioned free weight. They have been around for a long time but have resurfaced as a prime exercise tool, especially for core exercises. Some are hard and bounce like a basketball; some are soft and don't bounce at all. What matters is how much the medicine ball weighs (between 10 and 15 pounds is best) and its size (which should be about the size of a basketball or volleyball). The medicine ball is heavy compared to most sport balls, but you won't be kicking or throwing it for any distance, and the weight of the ball is its greatest benefit. It provides resistance in an unusual form. Although it's a little ungainly and takes some practice to control, once you get the hang of it, it's fun and very effective.

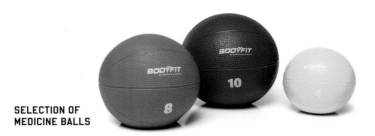

**SELECTION OF
MEDICINE BALLS**

Ankle Weights

Ankle weights are often overlooked as a source of resistance. By strapping an ankle weight around your leg just above your foot, you increase your body weight by that amount. You can get ankle weights that are adjustable, usually from 1 to 10 pounds, so you have some room to increase the resistance over time. Any exercise that involves lifting your legs off the floor—the walking lunge, step-up, or lying leg lift, for example—can be made a little more challenging with an ankle weight.

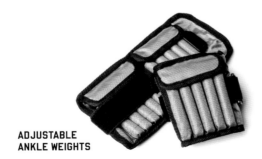

**ADJUSTABLE
ANKLE WEIGHTS**

The gym is likely to have all of this equipment, but there are a lot of exercises that can be done at home if you choose to simply invest in resistance bands, a couple sets of dumbbells or a medicine ball, and an exercise ball. This type of equipment is also very light (except for heavier dumbbells and medicine balls) and doesn't take up much space, so it's also very handy when traveling. Appendix B lists the exercises that are most accessible at home or while traveling.

CHAPTER 5

Warm-up, Cooldown, and Flexibility

Proper warm-up, cooldown, and flexibility add to the effectiveness of training by preparing your body for work, helping your body recover from the workout, and making sure you can move through the proper range of motion. Quite often the warm-up, cooldown, and flexibility portions of a workout are minimized or completely ignored. A training program is only complete if every component is sufficiently included. There are many physiological benefits to warming up before exercise, some life-saving reasons to cool down after a workout, and lots of stress reduction to be found in a flexibility program. This chapter details some of the truths and myths about these training components and provides the knowledge you need to put together a well-rounded program.

Getting Your Body Ready

As a dedicated triathlete, you wouldn't get out of bed in the morning, put on your running shoes, and hit the road without warming up. If you have been around triathlons for any time, you have seen other athletes doing a few laps in the pool or lake, riding their bikes, or jogging around the transition area. They do this to better prepare their bodies for the challenges ahead. Warming up has long been a part of an endurance athlete's preparations, but when it comes to strength training, it is often misunderstood.

There are a couple of typical claims about what a warm-up does to help prepare the body to lift weights: that it increases blood flow to the muscles, and that it increases the muscle temperature. While these points are true, that's not the end of the story. Warm-ups for cardio exercise and for resistance exercise are a little different. Typical cardio exercise is done for several minutes continuously, so these benefits do occur. However, a traditional strength training warm-up is usually done by completing one or two sets of an exercise with a really light weight before completing the assigned sets and repetitions with a normal weight. These extra sets only take a minute or two, with some rest in between and then more rest before starting the real workout. As a result of these rest periods, the increases in blood flow and muscle temperature are not retained. The body responds to exercise by increasing blood flow to the working muscles, but when work stops, blood flow to those muscles is reduced very quickly. Because it takes continuous work (in the range of 10 minutes) to increase muscle temperature, doing a couple of short sets does not help.

Another reason often given for completing light warm-up sets is that it alerts the central nervous system by simulating the work about to be done and allows the brain to start sending the correct motor pattern signals to the muscles. This is true; however, research hasn't shown that warm-up sets have any physiological benefit, and you would need to do a warm-up before each exercise, thus adding a lot of time to your workout that doesn't provide you any proven benefit.

Instead of starting your strength workouts with traditional warm-up sets, complete a short warm-up on a cardio machine that uses both the upper- and lower-body muscles. Examples are light jogging on a treadmill without holding on (your arms have to work), using a rowing machine, or using an elliptical machine or bike that has moving arm handles. Any of these will get blood flowing to all of the muscles in your limbs, and after about 10 to 15 minutes, your muscle temperature will rise as well. A higher muscle temperature allows the energy processes to work faster, leads to faster removal of by-products such as lactate, and creates quicker muscle contractions.

If you still want to do a light warm-up set before your heavier lifting, go directly to the exercise, do a light warm-up, and then immediately start your regular routine. After you start your workout, your body may cool back down between sets, but not very much. Your heart rate won't return to resting, so you will be pumping blood to the muscles much more quickly as long as you are working out. The short rests between sets will cause a small reduction in blood flow and temperature, but the initial elevation will help carry you through your workout. The key is to limit your rest time between sets as much as possible. This is where grouping your exercises so that you can work one area while another is resting helps maintain blood flow and temperature. Even walking around in between sets is better than sitting and waiting for the next set. As long as you keep moving, your body will stay warmed up and ready to exercise.

Workout Recovery

Your body does not go right back to its resting level immediately after cessation of exercise. Heart rate and ventilation remain at a higher level for a short time while your body continues to remove metabolic by-products from muscle, replenish energy stores, and reduce

▰ One of the most important reasons to COOL DOWN is to prevent blood pooling in the legs.

body temperature. As part of your cardio training, you may exercise at a low intensity to cool down, or you may take a short walk until your heart rate returns to resting and you have stopped sweating. In strength training, you need to aim for the same objectives.

One of the most important reasons to cool down is to prevent blood pooling in the legs. During exercise, the heart pumps blood down to the legs (with the help of gravity), and the contractions of leg muscles push blood back to the heart to be recirculated. The heart is a great pump, but it's only good at pushing blood out, not sucking it back in—that requires a "muscle pump," which only works if you are moving. If you stop moving, the extra blood that was sent to the muscles during exercise doesn't make its way back to the heart fast enough, and the heart has to work harder—keeping the heart rate higher for longer. In extreme circumstances, such as very hard training, exercising in the heat, or training only the lower-body muscles, this pooling can reduce the blood return to the heart so much that it puts excessive strain on the heart.

Cooling down can be simply walking around until your heart rate returns to near resting or doing just about any light cardio exercise. You should start your cooldown immediately after your last set and continue for as long as it takes to get your heart rate and breathing back to near resting. How long this takes will vary with the intensity of your workout (a hard workout takes longer to cool down from). The cooldown can be focused on lower-body exercise, such as walking, light jogging, or cycling, because gravity will help circulate the blood pumped to the upper body back to the heart. Stretching and flexibility training are *not* considered a cooldown—especially static stretching. Movement makes the "muscle pump" work, and static stretching or sitting down isn't moving, so they are not effective cooldowns.

Stretch to Move

Stretching has long been touted as an important component of any fitness program. Flexibility is the ability to move the body in a wide range of purposeful movements at a required speed. It determines how we move. If your body is not capable of moving through the range of motion required for an exercise, you can't do that exercise properly. Likewise, if you cannot move through a particular range of motion at the speed required for an exercise, you can't do that exercise properly. If an exercise movement is difficult and makes you feel like you are being stretched, that is because you lack the flexibility you need to move through the required range of motion. The exercise movement should never be difficult to do or seem like a stretch in itself.

During strength training you should always be able to complete an entire movement with ease—meaning you don't have to force your body into a particular position or through a particular movement. If you are not flexible enough, you will compensate by allowing another body part to relax and move, thus losing correct technique. For example, if your calf muscles are too tight, a squat exercise presents a difficult range of movement. You will likely alter the exercise technique by lifting your heels so you can continue to squat down to the required position. Instead of doing the exercise correctly, you compromise technique and position yourself for injury. The solution is to improve your flexibility. An exercise is only dangerous when it's done incorrectly, and not being flexible enough to maintain correct technique is just plain dangerous. A proper stretching program will allow you to move through the required range of motion for any exercise.

Stretching has long been described as a means to reduce soreness, but there is no research to support this claim. Soreness is mainly the result of eccentric contractions that occur when you are lowering a weight after a rep, and is a signal that some small amount of damage has been done. You will remain sore until the damage is repaired. Fortunately, soreness is usually temporary. No amount of stretching will make you less sore because stretching does not repair the damage. It may make you less tight, which makes it easier to move, but it will not cure injury.

Likewise, stretching is often listed as a way to prevent injury in general or during competition, but there is no evidence to support that either. Research has shown that the quantity and variety of injuries suffered by athletes in many different sports are the same whether they stretch or not. However, the benefit of proper flexibility is that it will allow you to move through a range of motion with ease, which will prevent you from getting hurt or straining your muscles and tendons.

You probably already do some sort of stretching along with your endurance training. If you find that you do not have the flexibility required to properly complete an exercise in your strength training program, make time to stretch each joint and muscle group that needs help. The only type of stretch shown to both increase and retain flexibility is static stretching. Each static stretch must be held from 30 to 60 seconds. There are dozens of different stretches, so seek out the ones that will most benefit you. A certified personal trainer or triathlon coach can make recommendations, or there are many online resources that describe different stretches.

Flexibility is something that everyone can improve upon, even if that improvement comes slowly. Stretching should follow the same rules as progression for strength training: If you progressively

■■■ Flexibility is something that everyone can improve upon, even if that IMPROVEMENT comes slowly.

stretch a little farther than you did before, you will increase your flexibility over time. Some muscles respond quickly and show great improvement, while others seem to barely move. But you won't see any improvement if you don't stretch, so no matter how little benefit you see, keep going—it will happen. Just like strength or endurance training, the benefit you get from stretching will be lost if you don't do it regularly. At the very least, stretch every other day to maintain your flexibility and range of motion.

Deciding how far you should stretch is always subjective, but a general rule to follow is to stretch into the uncomfortable zone, but not to the point of pain. You should feel a stretch, but it shouldn't hurt. The uncomfortable feeling of a stretch should go away as soon as you stop stretching; if it doesn't, then you went too far. It is better to let your body adjust slowly rather than to push hard just to try to get that extra little bit. Muscles will tear during a stretch, so you have to be careful, listen to your body, and know your limitations. Injuries during stretching are rare, but they do happen.

CHAPTER 6

Choosing Your Exercises and Order

Now that you understand the components of a total strength training program, you can design a workout for your needs. This chapter will help you choose the exercises that are best for you and arrange them in your workout. One of the best things about strength training is that there are very few rules that are carved in stone, so you can test several different approaches. There will probably be a lot of trial and a little error, so experiment until you find what works for you.

Which Exercises Fit You Best?

There are literally hundreds of different exercises, not all of them right for a triathlete. Chapters 8 through 14 feature the best exercises for triathletes, most of which focus specifically on the movements and positions involved in training and competition, along with several that train the body outside of triathlon-specific moves but provide a stronger base to work from. With so many exercises to choose from, completing all of them in a single training session just isn't possible. Evaluating your personal strengths and weaknesses during

TABLE 6.1. **STRENGTH TRAINING NEEDS ANALYSIS**

	SWIMMING
SYMPTOM: You have to rest your legs periodically and rely more on your arms. **CAUSE:** Relatively weak lower body	**SOLUTION:** Strengthen your quads, glutes, and hips.
SYMPTOM: You have to kick harder at times to let your arms rest. **CAUSE:** Relatively weak upper body	**SOLUTION:** Strengthen your shoulders, arms, and back.
SYMPTOM: Your body roll decreases the farther or longer you swim. **CAUSE:** Core muscle fatigue	**SOLUTION:** Add core exercises that work on rotation.
SYMPTOM: One leg becomes more tired than the other. **CAUSE:** Muscular imbalance in legs	**SOLUTION:** Incorporate more single-leg exercises.
SYMPTOM: One arm or shoulder becomes more tired than the other. **CAUSE:** Muscular imbalance in arms/shoulders	**SOLUTION:** Incorporate more single-arm exercises.
SYMPTOM: You sometimes have to increase your stroke rate to maintain the same speed. **CAUSE:** Not enough muscular endurance and weak upper body	**SOLUTION:** Increase reps and the number of upper-body exercises.

and after training will lead you to the best exercises to improve your performances. Table 6.1 presents a strength training needs analysis to help you discover what areas your strength program should concentrate on. Use those answers to guide you to the Exercise Index (Appendix A), which will recommend specific exercises for each muscle group and event.

To figure out your areas of weakness, look at each portion of your triathlon training individually (swim, bike, and run), then in pairs (swim-bike and bike-run), and then as a complete set. Analyzing your fatigue, aches and pains, or weakness during and after each event will help you understand which muscles need more work, which will then point you in the direction of the best exercises to

	CYCLING
SYMPTOM: You push harder with one leg or the other. **CAUSE:** Muscular imbalance in legs	**SOLUTION:** Use more weight on single-leg exercises for your weak side.
SYMPTOM: Your thighs start to become tired before your hips and glutes do. **CAUSE:** Weak quadriceps	**SOLUTION:** Incorporate more exercises that extend your knee.
SYMPTOM: Your heels start to drop below your toes as you push on the pedals. **CAUSE:** Weak calf muscles	**SOLUTION:** Add more calf raises, step-ups, and walking lunges.
SYMPTOM: Your arms or shoulders become fatigued if you don't use aerobars. **CAUSE:** Weak shoulders and/or arms	**SOLUTION:** Train your shoulders and triceps more.
SYMPTOM: Your shoulders or upper back become fatigued while using aerobars. **CAUSE:** Weak shoulders and/or upper back	**SOLUTION:** Strengthen your shoulders and upper back.
SYMPTOM: Your back sags instead of staying flat. **CAUSE:** Weak upper and lower back	**SOLUTION:** Include more core exercises that strengthen your back.

Continued

include in your program. For each individual event, ask yourself which muscle groups feel the most fatigued or feel weaker than the others, or if a particular area of your body or muscle group becomes noticeably sore during or immediately after training or remains sore for longer than others. Focus your strength training on these areas.

When you complete endurance training in bricks, or pairs (swim-bike or bike-run), analyze how each muscle group feels during the second event, after it has already been worked during the first event. For example, how do your legs feel during the bike after your swim compared to how they feel during the bike when you don't swim first? If there is a big difference, you may need to spend more time training your legs to be stronger during the swim so they won't

TABLE 6.1. **STRENGTH TRAINING NEEDS ANALYSIS** CONTINUED

RUNNING	
SYMPTOM: You drag your toes. **CAUSE:** Weak shin muscles	**SOLUTION:** Strengthen your dorsiflexor muscles.
SYMPTOM: Your hamstrings become tired before your quads do. **CAUSE:** Muscle imbalance in thighs	**SOLUTION:** Include more hamstring exercises.
SYMPTOM: Your quads become tired before your hamstrings do. **CAUSE:** Muscle imbalance in thighs	**SOLUTION:** Include more thigh exercises.
SYMPTOM: Your arms drop lower during long runs. **CAUSE:** Biceps fatigue	**SOLUTION:** Add more biceps exercises and reps.
SYMPTOM: Your shoulders become tight or start to hurt. **CAUSE:** Bouncing and fatiguing shoulders	**SOLUTION:** Focus more on shoulder strength for running.
SYMPTOM: You find yourself leaning forward. **CAUSE:** Lower back fatigue	**SOLUTION:** Include more upright core exercises.
SYMPTOM: Your strides become shorter as you run longer. **CAUSE:** Hip and glute fatigue	**SOLUTION:** Increase exercises for your hip and the range of motion used.

be so fatigued during the ride. Or, if your upper body is significantly more tired while running when you bike first, try working more on upper-body exercises for the bike.

Finally, analyze how your body feels after completing a triathlon, focusing on which muscles are the most fatigued and which are the sorest in the days following the competition. It is a common mistake to think that the legs are automatically the most fatigued because they are used the most during the last two events. If your shoulders are the most fatigued and sore, they need more work.

Another way to look at this is to evaluate when during a race you start feeling fatigued. For instance, you may feel really strong during the swim, but after the bike you slow down and lose power, so when it comes time to run, that is the most difficult. This indicates that you need to focus your strength training initially on improving your ability to swim and bike so that you aren't so fatigued when they are done. Then you will have more left for the run.

Ideally there will be time in your schedule to train every muscle group equally, but focusing on your weaknesses first is very important. If you start out by training everything, both your strong and your weak muscles will become stronger, but there will still be an imbalance; the strong become stronger while the weak just become strong. You should choose exercises that address your weaknesses and bring those muscles up to par with the rest of your body. Then you can start training everything.

In some cases, you may not be able to identify a particular weakness or training need. In this case, simply design your program to cover a little bit of everything: upper- and lower-body exercises for each event. Over time, every program should reach this point, so if you are there already, great—but there is always room for improvement, and you should remain open to identifying specific weaknesses or needs as your training progresses.

There are many ways to choose which groups of exercises you need to do, and your focus will change as you make improvements, so reevaluation is essential. However, don't constantly change your program in an effort to find the right exercises. You have to let your body adapt before altering the program again. A good rule of thumb is to give yourself six to eight weeks before rearranging your exercises so that you can really tell whether your body is responding. Also remember that change is going to take place on the inside, so don't judge your results by what you see in the mirror. Listen to and feel your body as you train. If you are not as fatigued as before, everything is probably working fine, so don't try to change it right away.

Find the exercises that stimulate your body to change positively and keep them in your program.

You really should enjoy the exercises you do. There is nothing worse than designing a program that you think will work but that you hate doing. Odds are you won't put 100 percent effort into it, won't focus on the exercises, and will put off training as much as possible. There is a saying that the exercises you dislike the most are the ones you need the most. Although there is some truth to this, the other side of the coin is that you have to like training. A compromise may be to introduce exercises that you don't particularly care for one at a time. Give yourself an opportunity to get used to them and see how they make your body change. Don't load up on a lot of hard exercises that make you look for ways out of training. Strike a balance—you can choose exercises just because you like them, but don't ignore what your body needs.

A word of caution: Any exercise that may cause a previous injury to flare up again should be avoided. For instance, if you have had an ACL injury, the leg extension exercise will place too much stress on your knee, so you should leave it out of your program. It is always a good idea to consult with a sports medicine physician if you are not sure whether an exercise could be problematic for you.

Selecting a Mix of Exercises

To determine how many exercises you can finish in a single session, aim for 6 to 10 from a combination of different muscles and events. Be sure to factor in how much time you have to train. If time is a constraint, focus on the most important exercises first, and if there is time left over, move down your list to other exercises. Allow more time for single-arm and single-leg exercises.

Once you define what you hope to accomplish with your strength program, you will be ready to review the selection of exercises in Part III. The exercises in Chapter 8 cover the core, and Chapters 9 through 14 are divided into upper-body and lower-body exercises for each event (swim, bike, and run). The upper body includes anything above the waist, and the lower body is everything below the waist. Your core is essentially everything from your hips to your neck, or everything except your head, arms, and legs.

It is not a good idea to do every exercise in a section; that will definitely cause overtraining and decrease your performance. In a perfect world, you should be able to do one exercise for each muscle and get everything you need from it. However, our bodies are a little more complicated than that, because each muscle contributes and moves in several different ways depending on which event you are focusing on. All the exercises for each muscle group are not the same and thus not strictly interchangeable; for example, the triceps push-down and the tubing kickback are both triceps exercises, but they work the triceps in different ways and have subtly different results.

A good rule to follow is to never do more than three exercises for any one muscle group during a single training session. You can choose three exercises from one event, or you can mix and match from two or three events, depending on what you need to accomplish. In addition, you should give a muscle time to recover after training, so never use the same exercises on two consecutive days. You can train the same muscle if you are not sore from the previous day's training, but use different exercises. This is an advanced way of training on consecutive days, and it must be approached with caution and by paying very close attention to your body's responses and levels of fatigue and soreness.

Exercise Program Rules

1 Do NOT perform every exercise in a session during one workout.

2 No more than 3 exercises for a muscle group (e.g., biceps or hamstrings).

3 Do NOT perform the same exercises on consecutive days. You can train the same muscles, but use different exercises.

4 Aim for 6 to 10 exercises per session.

5 Allow 6 to 8 weeks before changing the exercise program.

Exercise Order

The order in which you complete your exercises will have a substantial impact on the effectiveness of each exercise and the workout in general. There are several approaches to exercise order, each based on sound science, but none has been shown to be significantly better than another. Try changing up the exercise order from time to time, both to add variety to your workout and to create a new stimulus. It's a simple change, but it can provide just enough stimulus to keep your body adapting and growing stronger.

To illustrate this point, consider how the same set of exercises can be rearranged in each of the ways mentioned below. These eight exercises don't fit every exercise order perfectly, but the program you choose may not fit each scenario perfectly either. If the order you like best doesn't work perfectly with the exercises you have chosen, it's okay to do a variation on a couple of orders in a single workout, too. Remember that there are no hard-and-fast rules—just find something that works well for your goals.

Goal-Oriented Order

The first exercise order places the emphasis on those areas that you feel need the most work. In this case, you will order each exercise in your workout according to how important it is to your overall program goals. For example, if you feel that during the swim your shoulders are fatiguing too fast and are therefore a weak link, the exercises focusing on shoulder development for swimming should be the first ones you do. During a training session, this allows you to work the areas of emphasis while you are fresh and full of energy. Later in the session, as you are getting tired, is not the time to try to work what you feel to be the most important area. The exercises here are ordered to first work the shoulders and chest:

Dip	*delts, pecs, triceps*
Dumbbell Fly	*delts, pecs*
Tubing Row	*biceps, delts, lats*
Dumbbell Handle Push-up	*delts, pecs, triceps*
Moguls	*core*
Lateral Lunge	*glutes, hamstrings, quads*
Single-Leg Extension	*quads*
Squat	*calves, glutes, hamstrings, quads*

Big-Before-Small Order

The next order arranges exercises according to the size of the muscle(s) being worked. Larger muscles require more energy, so they should be trained before fatigue sets in. For example, squats would come before leg extensions, followed by the seated toe raise. This ensures that the most fatiguing exercises are done first. Those exercises that involve relatively smaller muscle groups are saved for last because they require less energy production. This style of order is based on the speed of metabolic energy depletion and restoration. During strength training, the main energy system is the ATP-PC (adenosine triphosphate–phosphocreatine) system, which supplies you with almost immediate energy to the muscles but lasts only about 10 seconds. When this is used up, the body relies on glycolysis to start converting stored glycogen to energy. This system lasts up to about two minutes. By that time you should have finished your set. Of key importance is not how fast these systems provide energy, but how fast they recover. It takes several minutes for the ATP-PC system to recover, so using it for the large muscle groups makes the most sense, as shown in this lineup of exercises:

Squat................................*calves, glutes, hamstrings, quads*
Dumbbell Handle Push-up................*delts, pecs, triceps*
Moguls..*core*
Lateral Lunge................*glutes, hamstrings, quads*
Dip................................*delts, pecs, triceps*
Tubing Row................*biceps, delts, lats*
Dumbbell Fly................*delts, pecs*
Single-Leg Extension................*quads*

Hard-to-Easy Order

This exercise order is subjective, being based on psychology rather than physiology. If you start your workout with the most difficult exercises rather than leaving them for last, you will be more likely to finish everything on your list. At one time or another, everyone has found a reason to skip out on the last part of a workout. Whatever the reason, skipping the hard exercise just makes it that much more difficult the next time. The less often you do an exercise, the slower your body will improve and adapt, which delays your performance progress. Doing a hard exercise first and getting it out of the way makes it much easier to complete the simple exercises. This sample order moves from difficult to easier movements:

Squat..*difficult*
Dip...*difficult*
Moguls...*difficult*
Dumbbell Handle Push-up...............................*moderate*
Dumbbell Fly...*moderate*
Tubing Row..*easier*
Lateral Lunge...*easier*
Single-Leg Extension...*easier*

Multiple-Joint-to-Single-Joint Order

Arranging your exercises based on how many joints are involved is similar to arranging them based on muscle size. The more joints that are involved, the more muscle is involved. More joints moving during an exercise also makes the exercise more complicated, and controlling technique more difficult. It takes more focus and technique to do a tubing stroke exercise, which involves three joints, than to do a triceps pushdown, which only involves a single joint. Because proper technique is key to preventing injury and getting the most out of an exercise, it follows that those exercises that involve the most complicated maneuvers should be done on the front end of a workout, as shown here:

Squat...*multiple joint*
Moguls..*multiple joint*
Lateral Lunge..*multiple joint*
Tubing Row...*multiple joint*
Dip..*multiple joint*
Dumbbell Handle Push-up.....................*multiple joint*
Single-Leg Extension....................................*single joint*
Dumbbell Fly..*single joint*

Upper-and-Lower-Body Alternating Order

Previous chapters discussed arranging exercises so that you could allow one body part to rest while another worked. One way of accomplishing this is by alternating upper-body and lower-body exercises. For the most part, these exercises are independent of each other. The only case in which they overlap is where the lower body supports the upper-body exercise while standing, which doesn't add much work to the lower body unless you just finished a difficult lower-body exercise and those muscles are fatigued. Switching between upper- and lower-body exercises, as shown in this list, offers the added advantage of keeping your heart pumping blood to different areas:

Dumbbell Handle Push-up..*upper*
Squat..*lower*
Dip..*upper*
Lateral Lunge...*lower*
Tubing Row..*upper*
Single-Leg Extension...*lower*
Dumbbell Fly...*upper*
Moguls...*core*

Push-Pull Alternating Order

Another way of alternating exercises is by doing one push, then one pull exercise. A push exercise is any action in which you are pushing a weight away from you (e.g., leg press, dumbbell shoulder press, triceps push-down). A pull exercise brings the weight closer to you (e.g., dumbbell curl, lying leg curl, bridging pullover). Not every exercise will clearly fall into a push or pull category (e.g., walking lunge, back extension, split squat), so this becomes a little fuzzy now and then. The basis for push-pull is that opposing muscle groups can be worked in order. For example, alternating a set of dumbbell curls with a set of dips works both sides of the arms, so while the biceps are resting, the triceps work. Combining push-pull in an organization of opposing muscle groups is the most effective way to work this exercise order:

Dumbbell Fly	*push*
Tubing Row	*pull*
Squat	*push*
Moguls	*pull*
Dip	*push*
Lateral Lunge	*pull*
Dumbbell Handle Push-up	*push*
Single-Leg Extension	*push*

As mentioned earlier, your choice of exercises may not fit one or more of these exercise orders perfectly, but that's okay; you can make up a new exercise order to fit your program and your needs. For example, you may use half of your exercises in a goal-oriented order and half in a push-pull order. Or maybe you have a couple of hard exercises you want to get done first, then finish the rest in an alternating upper- and lower-body order. Any way you design your workout, the order has to fit what you want to achieve and may not align perfectly with these examples or any other exercise order you read about. The point is to make sure that your body's needs are put first and foremost in order to get the biggest benefit from your training.

CHAPTER 7

Sample Training Programs

There is no single strength training program that will fit every triathlete. Likewise, there are countless possibilities for how to shape a strength training program, so it's not possible to include all of them here. Instead, this chapter provides an idea of the types of programs you can design based on the length of triathlon you are training for, any deficiencies you are working to overcome, and different exercise orders. There are circuit programs and periodized programs, as well as general strength programs. Any of them can be oriented toward improving muscular endurance, hypertrophy, strength, or power.

These sample programs are based on the actual training practices of athletes, but that doesn't mean you should use them exactly as they are presented here. There is no guarantee they will work for you, because they were not designed for you. Look at how they are put together and substitute exercises you have chosen and workloads that are appropriate for your body to develop a program that will take you to new levels of performance.

Sprint Distance

Sprint triathlons are more about speed than about endurance. You need cardiovascular endurance, but because the distances are shorter, you don't have to pace yourself for as long, and you can compete at a higher intensity. With higher cardiovascular intensity comes the need for more muscular power (the ability of muscles to contract very fast). In addition, because sprint triathlons are the shortest, you may be more likely to compete in a greater number of competitions per season, so you will need a strength training program that takes that into account. Following are a few possible workout designs that are very effective for sprint distances.

Circuit Program for Sprint-Distance Triathletes

A circuit program will have very short rest intervals between each exercise—basically only as long as it takes to get to the next exercise. Instead of completing all of the sets of an exercise before moving on to the next one, you will complete one set of each exercise in your workout, then repeat the circuit until you have finished all your sets. The order of your exercises is up to you, but alternating muscle groups is the most practical choice. A circuit of 6 to 10 exercises will only take about 30 minutes to complete. You can design several different circuits so that you have a different workout every day, or use the same one each time, as long as you allow enough rest time so your muscles are fully recovered from the last workout. What follows are two different circuit workouts for a sprint distance triathlete: one focuses on building strength and power for cycling, and the other builds upper-body endurance for running and swimming.

Circuit Program to Improve Strength and Power in Cycling

Program Overview

GOAL	% 1RM	SETS	REPS
Strength and Power	85	3	6

Workout Instructions

Complete 1 set of each exercise in order, resting only long enough to move to the next exercise. Repeat circuit until all 3 sets are complete.

Workout Circuit

Step-up
Dumbbell Incline Press
Dumbbell Deep Squat
Shoulder Dip
Knee Raise
Back Extension
Seated Leg Curl
Barbell Front Raise

Workout moves from multijoint to single-joint exercises, alternating lower and upper body.

Circuit Program to Improve Upper-Body Muscular Endurance for Running and Swimming

Program Overview

GOAL	% 1RM	SETS	REPS
Muscular Endurance	70	2	12

Workout Instructions

Complete 1 set of each exercise in the first circuit, resting only long enough to move to the next exercise. Repeat the circuit for a second set. Using the same method, do 2 sets of each exercise in the second circuit.

Workout Circuit 1
Barbell Lift
Barbell Row
Hammer Curl
Dumbbell French Curl

Workout Circuit 2
Dumbbell Front Raise
Dumbbell Shoulder Press
Tubing Kickback
Dumbbell Curl

Workout is a double circuit. Each circuit begins with goal-oriented exercises that focus on the shoulders.

Periodization Program for Sprint-Distance Triathletes

Because several sprint triathlons can be completed in a single season, a periodized plan for the sprint athlete will not require large amounts of time. The cycles will be short and the entire plan will be repeated between events. A six-week periodization will provide enough time for two to three mesocycles to be completed, with microcycles only lasting one week. This means that you have to be prepared to change

Periodization Program Targeting Strength for Swimming

Program Overview

GOAL	WEEK	% 1RM	SETS	REPS
Muscular Endurance (Mesocycle 1)	1	62	3	18
	2	67	3	15
Hypertrophy (Mesocycle 2)	3	75	4	10
	4	80	4	8
Strength (Mesocycle 3)	5	85	4	6
	6	90	4	4

Workout Instructions

Complete 1 set of each exercise in the circuit, then finish all sets before moving to the next circuit.

Workout Circuit 1

Leg Extension
Lying Leg Curl
Cable Lateral Lift
Seated Calf Raise

} *Lower-body circuit works big muscles, then smaller muscles.*

Workout Circuit 2

Tubing Stroke
Dumbbell Shoulder Press
Bridging Pullover
One-Arm Throw
Dumbbell Curl

} *Upper-body circuit works big muscles, then smaller muscles.*

Periodization Program Targeting Hypertrophy for Improved Running

Program Overview

GOAL	WEEK	% 1RM	SETS	REPS
Muscular Endurance (Mesocycle 1)	1	55	3	15
	2	60	3	12
	3	65	2	15
Hypertrophy (Mesocycle 2)	4	70	4	12
	5	75	4	10
	6	80	3	10

Workout Instructions, Weeks 1–3

Complete 1 set of each pair of exercises, finishing all sets before moving to the next pair of exercises. Rest 30 seconds between sets.

3 Workout Circuits

Lateral Raise
Hammer Curl

Squat
Standing Leg Curl

Runner's Raise
Tubing Row

Each pair includes a push and a pull exercise.

Workout Instructions, Weeks 4–6

Complete 1 set of each exercise, then repeat circuit until sets are done.

Workout Circuit

Split Squat
Lying Single-Leg Curl
Upright Row
Shrug
Leg Press
Cable Hip Flex

Exercises alternate push and pull, upper and lower body.

your intensity and volume every week, but not necessarily your exercises. You can opt to keep the same exercises for the entire macrocycle and only change them when you start a new macrocycle, or you can change exercises in each mesocycle. In the two sample periodized programs, one contains two mesocycles with different exercises (page 85), and the other contains three mesocycles with the same exercises but more changes in goal and intensity or volume (page 84).

All-Around Program for Sprint-Distance Triathletes

If you don't have a particular muscular deficiency to work on, a good general workout can be used with either the 2-for-2 Rule or circular progression. There's no limit to the different sequences of exercises that you can design. All-around workouts pull from every discipline, both upper and lower body, and typically focus on exercises that are multijoint so that several muscle groups are worked simultaneously. The sample all-around program provides examples of such workouts.

SPRINT

All-Around Program for Swimming, Cycling, and Running

Program Overview
The following workouts can be used with the 2-for-2 Rule or circular progression plans, and with any combination of sets, reps, and intensity (% 1RM).

Workout Circuit 1	**Workout Circuit 2**	
Dip	Bridging Pullover	
Lateral Lunge	Inclined Superman	*Both workouts include*
Dumbbell Handle Push-up	Dumbbell Incline Press	*multijoint exercises,*
Step-up	Reverse Lunge	*alternating upper and*
Dumbbell Upright Row	Runner's Raise	*lower body.*
Squat	Dumbbell Split Squat	

Olympic Distance

Olympic-distance triathlons require more endurance than sprint-distance triathlons, but there is still an emphasis on speed. Because of the longer distances, the triathlete's muscles must be able to handle much more repetition and still provide the necessary force to keep them moving forward. Fewer Olympic-distance triathlons are typically completed in a season than sprint-distance triathlons, so the amount of training in between events is greater and takes place over a longer period of time. Periodized plans fit better with Olympic-distance racing because more time can be spent in each microcycle, allowing the body to adapt more before moving on to the next microcycle or mesocycle. Circuit programs also work and allow a triathlete to change his or her workout as often as desired with little planning.

Circuit Program for Olympic-Distance Triathletes

Either circular progression or the 2-for-2 Rule can be effectively used with a circuit program for Olympic-distance-triathlon strength training. The use of more than one circuit allows more variety and a greater training frequency (more days per week). A sample program on page 88 shows how you can use two circuits that train different body parts on consecutive days. A second program option, on page 89, shows how to train the same body part on consecutive days with different exercises, although this is more advanced and should be used only after considerable training experience.

Circuit Program to Improve Muscular Endurance for Cycling and Strength for Running

Program Overview

GOAL	% 1RM	SETS	REPS
Muscular Endurance/Cycling			
Upper-Body Circuit	65	3	15
Lower-Body Circuit	67	3	12
Strength/Running			
Lower-Body Circuit	87	4	6
Upper-Body Circuit	90	3	6

Workout Instructions

Complete 1 set of each exercise in each circuit, then repeat until all sets are complete.

Day 1 Running Lower-Body Circuit
Leg Press
Cable Hip Flex
Dumbbell Split Squat
Seated Toe Raise
Standing Leg Curl

Each circuit moves from multijoint to single-joint exercises.

Day 1 Cycling Upper-Body Circuit
Dumbbell Handle Push-up
Shoulder Dip
Dumbbell Incline Press
Barbell Front Raise

Note: You will complete 4 sets of the running lower-body circuit, beginning and ending with this lower-body circuit.

Day 2 Cycling Lower-Body Circuit
Walking Lunge
One-Leg Squat
Knee Raise
Seated Leg Curl
Single-Calf Raise

Each circuit moves from multijoint to single-joint exercises.

Day 2 Running Upper-Body Circuit
Upright Row
Tubing Row
Retraction
Shrug

Circuit Program Targeting Hypertrophy for Swimming

Program Overview

GOAL	%1RM	SETS	REPS
Hypertrophy	70	4	10

Workout Instructions

Complete 1 set of each exercise in the circuit, then repeat circuit until all sets are complete. Rest only long enough to get to the next exercise.

Day 1 Circuit
Dumbbell Shoulder Press
Tubing Kickback
Leg Extension
Standing Calf Raise
One-Arm Throw
Slam Dunk
Cable Lateral Lift
Inclined Superman

Day 2 Circuit
Tubing Stroke
Dumbbell Angled Raise
Seated Calf Raise
Cable Hip Extension
Dumbbell Curl
Bridging Pullover
Cable Lateral Cross
Lying Leg Curl

Workouts alternate push and pull exercises.

Periodized Program for Olympic-Distance Triathletes

Periodized strength training programs for Olympic-distance triathlons take a little more time to plan because they are approximately twice as long as sprint-distance plans. This is good for the athlete who likes to spend more time adapting to a particular intensity of training before changing it up. In addition, the increase in the percentage of your 1-rep max from one microcycle to the next is smaller, so increases in weight are not as great a shock to the body. Finally, more mesocycles can be included, so more physiological goals can be focused on, although you do have the option of using only two mesocycles and goals, if you like. Two examples of a 12-week periodization plan are shown on pages 90–91 and 92–93. The first uses three mesocycles of differing lengths, with microcycles varying in length, intensity, and number of exercises. However, a periodized plan does not have to be this complicated; a complicated design doesn't yield any extra benefit. By using the same length of time for each mesocycle and microcycle and the same number of exercises, as shown in the second example, the plan can be greatly simplified, which makes it easier to remember, execute, and enjoy.

OLYMPIC

Periodization Program Targeting Strength for Swimming

Program Overview

GOAL	WEEK	% 1RM	SETS	REPS
Muscular Endurance (Mesocycle 1)	1	55	2	20
	2	57	2	18
	3–4	60	2	16
	5–6	65	2	14
Hypertrophy (Mesocycle 2)	7–8	70	3	10
	9–10	80	3	8
Strength (Mesocycle 3)	11	85	4	6
	12	95	6	2

Workout Instructions, Weeks 1–6
Complete all sets of each exercise before moving to next exercise. Rest 30 seconds between sets.

Workout Circuit
Dip
Squat
Slam Dunk
Leg Press
Hammer Curl
Lying Leg Curl
Bridging Pullover
Cable Hip Flex
Seated Toe Raise

Workout moves from hard to easy exercises.

Workout Instructions, Weeks 7–10

Complete 1 set of each exercise in the circuit, then repeat until all 3 sets are done. Rest between exercises only long enough to get to the next exercise.

Workout Circuit

Squat
Dumbbell Shoulder Press
Upright Row
Leg Extension
Cable Toe Raise
Tubing Kickback

Circuit moves from hard to easy exercises.

Workout Instructions, Weeks 11–12

Complete all sets of each exercise before moving to the next exercise. Rest 90 seconds between sets.

Workout Circuit

Squat
Leg Extension
Lying Leg Curl
Seated Calf Raise
Lateral Raise
Tubing Kickback
Shrug
Retraction

Workout moves from hard to easy exercises.

Periodization Program Targeting Strength for Cycling and Running

Program Overview

GOAL	WEEK	%1RM	SETS	REPS
Muscular Endurance	1–2	63	2	16
(Mesocycle 1)	3–4	67	2	14
Hypertrophy	5–6	70	3	10
(Mesocycle 2)	7–8	80	3	8
Strength	9–10	85	4	6
(Mesocycle 3)	11–12	95	6	2

Workout Instructions, Weeks 1–4

Complete 1 set of each exercise in the circuit, then repeat until both sets are done. Rest between exercises ony long enough to get to the next exercise.

Workout Circuit

Shoulder Dip
Reverse Dumbbell Curl
Triceps Pushdown   *Circuit works upper body,*
Dumbbell Split Squat   *then lower body.*
Cable Toe Raise
Romanian Deadlift

Workout Instructions, Weeks 5–8

Complete all sets of each exercise before moving to the next exercise. Rest 30 seconds between sets.

Workout Circuit

Hammer Curl
Shrug   *Exercises begin*
Barbell Row   *with upper body,*
Dumbbell Deep Squat   *then lower body.*
Seated Leg Curl
Knee Raise

> **Workout Instructions, Weeks 9–12**
> Complete all sets of each exercise before moving to the next exercise.
> Rest 90 seconds between sets.
>
> **Workout Circuit**
> Barbell Wrist Curl
> Upright Row
> Bench Press   *Circuit works upper*
> Lying Single-Leg Curl   *body, then lower body.*
> Single-Leg Extension
> Leg Press

Half-Iron to Iron Distance

The long-distance triathlons take the greatest toll on the body's energy and muscular systems. Although muscular endurance is key to completing this distance, strength, power, and hypertrophy have a place as well. Remember that you can either train for more muscular endurance or make your muscles bigger and then make those larger muscles stronger and more powerful, which will provide you with more endurance. Periodization is the best way to prepare for long-distance triathlons. Circuits built within a periodized program are part of the game plan, but the overall change in goals and training emphasis really prepares you for the event.

The program on page 94 is a sample plan to accompany six months of long-distance-triathlon training. If you don't plan to do more than two long-distance triathlons in a season, you can spend more time preparing for each. However, if you plan on competing in multiple long-distance events in a single season, you can either design your periodization plan similar to the shorter style described for the Olympic distance or stick with a longer plan that encompasses the event within it. For example, you could plan a six-month periodization plan but insert a tapering week and a race within it,

Periodization Program Targeting Strength for Triathlon

Program Overview

GOAL	WEEK	%1RM	SETS	REPS
Muscular Endurance (Mesocycle 1)	1–3	55	3	20
	4–6	58	3	18
	7–8	61	3	16
	9–10	63	2	20
	11–12	65	2	18
	13–14	67	2	16
Hypertrophy (Mesocycle 2)	15–17	72	3	10
	18–20	79	3	8
Strength (Mesocycle 3)	21–22	85	4	5
	23–24	88	4	4

Workout Instructions

Select a mix of exercises specific to swimming, cycling, and running, and order the workout to be goal-oriented by event. Add exercises as your training requires.

then after that week, pick back up the training where you left off. Good execution of a periodized plan depends on strength peaking right before your most important events. Inserting other less important events over the course of your strength training is fine.

Six months is really about the longest program you can design without a lot of guesswork, because it is difficult to estimate what you will be capable of doing beyond that time. The key to a successful long-term periodization plan is the testing. Initially, you must determine your 1-rep max for each exercise. Approximately halfway through the program, retest again and adjust the weights you are using. This will keep the stimulus accurate and your results coming.

Because this type of program is all-inclusive and can involve many different exercises, you can make each microcycle completely different from previous cycles. You can vary which exercises you use and how many you use, depending on how your cardio training is coming along. You only have to define the cycles, intensities, and sets or repetitions initially, then add the exercises as you go along. Remember that you really need to include as many as possible, if not all, of the different exercises to ensure that you cover every muscle group in every event and motion possible.

Finally, be prepared to stop and rewrite the program somewhere along the way. If you are unable to keep up with the increasing intensity and need more time in any single microcycle, that's just fine; adjust the rest of the program and keep going. The ability to make changes midstream is important to long-term planning. If you aren't flexible, you won't be able to maintain the level of training that you prescribed for yourself, and your performance will suffer.

Filling In the Gaps

Randomized Workout

If you go to a gym on a regular basis, you'll notice people who just randomly do different exercises, seemingly without any particular training program or goal in mind. If you are new to strength training, you will see results from doing this type of workout; but you would see results from just about anything that your body is not used to. Having a goal in mind, and a strength training program designed to meet that goal, is a much better solution. However, every once in awhile it is actually a good idea to give yourself a break from your regular program, especially if you find yourself less than enthusiastic about completing it that day. Additionally, not every conceivable exercise that you may benefit from is included in this book; that would require an encyclopedia-size text. You may find another exercise you like that fits your goals, or you may see a new piece of equipment at the gym and want to try it out—go ahead. Taking a day off from your regular workout now and then and just randomly trying some new exercises, or going back to an exercise you have done before, is fine. The body thrives on change and new workloads. Remember that overload is essential for making improvements in your strength. Overload can also come in the form of an exercise that is new and different from what you have been doing.

A randomized workout should not be an easy workout, so it should still challenge you in both intensity and volume. Since the exercise will be new to you, start with a light weight to perfect your form first, then increase it to a level that fits within the sets and reps range for your particular physiological goal (muscular endurance, hypertrophy, strength, or power). Use 6 to 10 random exercises, either from this book or new ones you find or that you see at the gym, to fill out a complete workout.

Core Workout

Core workouts consist of exercises like those found in Chapter 8. A core workout will differ from your other strength workouts in that the exercises do not use a specific percentage of your 1-rep max because they do not use much external weight. Instead, core exercises will use just body weight, resistance tubing, or a medicine ball. These exercises also include specific sets and reps recommendations, so building a core workout is really as simple as choosing what exercises you want to include. As a general rule, you should not do more than six core exercises in one workout. Each exercise will be using most of the same muscle groups and are mostly designed for muscular endurance training, so more than six exercises would make the program too intense and possibly cause some overtraining or injury. While all core exercises challenge the muscles in the torso, those that require external resistance will also work the arms and/or legs as well. Design your program by alternating exercises that add resistance using a medicine ball or resistance tubing, and exercises without external resistance. When you want to use two consecutive exercises that use resistance, alternate between the resistance tubing and a medicine ball. Below are two examples of a core workout.

Core Workout Example 1

Complete 1 set of each exercise in the circuit, then repeat for a second set.

Combination Crunch	20 reps
Diagonal Wood Chop	20 reps
Stability Ball Bridge	1 min.
Stump Throw	20 reps
Moguls	20 reps
Lunging Russian Twist	30 reps

Core Workout Example 2

Complete 1 set of each exercise in the circuit, repeat for a second set, then repeat the first three exercises for a third set.

Pendulum	20 reps
Two-Arm Throw	15 reps
Standing Russian Twist	20 reps
V-up	15 reps
Balanced Cross-Pull	15 reps
Modified Sit-up	10 reps

Travel Workout

Staying on your exercise plan and getting a decent workout while on the road can be difficult unless you plan ahead. Luckily, just about every town has a gym, so you always have the option of going as a guest or paying a small fee for a daily membership to keep yourself on track. This has the added bonus of exposing you to new equipment and possibly new ideas for your workout. You can also get an unexpected motivational bump when working out in a new gym while traveling. Something about being in a new setting gives you renewed energy to get in a really good workout that day. Also, don't forget about hotel fitness centers. These are typically very sparsely equipped, with a couple of cardio machines and some dumbbells, but they can provide ample space to do your workout.

Another option is to have a travel workout ready to go in these situations. You can design a workout based on your needs and goals using the exercises in this book that do not require any equipment, or just resistance tubing that can be easily packed in your suitcase (and left in there between trips so you never forget to pack it). Using the same parameters you have set for your typical workout, change the exercises as needed to keep your body working while you travel. In some cases the resistance provided by resistance tubing or body weight may not be as much as you are used to, so the workout may just train for muscular endurance. This is fine because it is still providing your muscles with some resistance, which will help keep you on track until you can return to your usual program.

If you need to shorten the workout due to time constraints, focus on your most important goals first, spending the majority of the time you have on those exercises. Travel is also a good time for those random workouts mentioned above. When you are traveling on family vacation or for business, you won't usually have a large block of free time except at the end of the day when you are typically exhausted already. In these cases you can split up your workout into smaller pieces, completing two to three exercises in the morning and maybe a couple more at night. Traveling can present challenges to a typical workout, so you have to be flexible and do what you can when you can. The key is that you stay on track. One or two days off can be good for rest and recuperation, but any longer and you start losing the progress you have made, so schedule in some workout time to keep your body progressing.

The travel workouts that follow are designed to stimulate each muscle group each day. They are split into two short workouts, but they can be combined if you have the time. One workout targets the core and upper body, the other hits the core and lower body. Each one utilizes exercises from each triathlon discipline, so there is a little something for everything. As mentioned before, you can alternate the exercises you need based on your goals to achieve the same type of workout; the possibilities are endless.

Travel Workout Examples

Complete the required number of sets and reps based on your goals.

Core/Upper-Body Exercises

V-up

Tubing Stroke

Dumbbell Handle Push-up

Tubing Row

Bridging Pullover

Core/Lower-Body Exercises

Combination Crunch

Lateral Lunge

One-Leg Squat

Cable Hip Flex

Toe Taps

PART III

EXERCISES

CHAPTER 8

Exercises for Core Conditioning

Core conditioning focuses on every muscle except those in your arms, legs, and head. Although you may move these body parts during core exercises, they won't be the main muscle groups getting a workout. *Core* has been defined as the abdominal muscles (abs) and lower back, but in fact it is the part of your body to which everything is attached and from which every movement is controlled—that is, your entire torso. Whether you are climbing into the pool, putting on your running shoes, or riding your bike, your core muscles are involved.

Core conditioning is also sometimes referred to as functional training because it involves working muscles that help you move the rest of your body. The surface muscles—those you can see in the mirror—are mostly responsible for the large movements; the following chapters cover them in detail. The deep core muscles help stabilize and control the surface muscles so that everything works together. Your core must be solid, otherwise you will use more energy to produce less-powerful movements.

This chapter focuses on a few of the many exercises that target the core. They were picked specifically because they work a lot of muscles very fast and very hard, in a manner that builds the best base for the triathlon-specific exercises in later chapters. Unlike many of the other exercises in this book, these core exercises include goal recommendations for repetitions and sets. Complete as many reps and sets in each exercise as you can do without pushing yourself to a point where the exercise becomes uncomfortable. Each exercise should be strenuous but should not cause pain. Many of these exercises also suggest a proper range of motion, but you should work within your personal range of motion and not push yourself too far too fast.

Core exercises do not use much external weight, and only a few use resistance tubing or a medicine ball, so you don't have to calculate what percentage of your 1-rep max to use. For those exercises that do require resistance tubing or a medicine ball, use one that allows you to complete the recommended reps and sets with enough resistance to make it challenging. As you get stronger, increase the intensity by increasing the weight of the medicine ball or the strength of the resistance tubing. The remainder of the exercises rely only on body weight and are used primarily to increase muscular endurance.

Finally, these core exercises do not focus on a single muscle group; each works the entire core, but each in a different way, so the results are different from one exercise to the next. While these exercises might not produce the kind of results you can see in the mirror, they do make a difference in your training and competition.

Combination Crunch

Lie faceup on a stability ball so that the top of the ball is positioned under the curve of your lower back, with your feet planted flat on the floor. Allow your body to arch backward over the ball. Lift your hips so they are at about the same height as your knees and move your feet away from the ball until they are directly under your knees. You can move your feet farther apart for more stability and balance or keep them close together for maximum instability (making the exercise harder). Cross your arms over your chest with your fingers touching your shoulders (see start).

Lift one of your shoulders up and across your body toward your opposite hip. At the same time, lift that opposite leg—the one you are crunching toward—and point it out and away from you (see midpoint). Immediately relax back to the start position and do a rep on the other side. Alternate reps from side to side until you have completed 20 reps, then rest for 30 seconds and do another set.

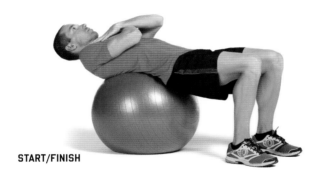

START/FINISH

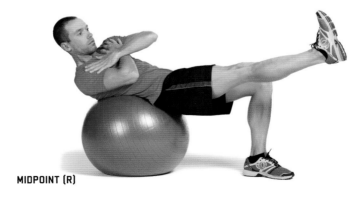

MIDPOINT (R)

V-up

Lie on your back with your feet and legs together and your arms extended over your head (see start). Clasp your hands together so your arms stay straight throughout the exercise.

Take a deep breath and slowly exhale while lifting your arms, upper body, and legs into the air, trying to bring them together as high as possible over your hips (see midpoint). When you get to the top of the movement, your entire upper body and legs should be off

the floor, with only your buttocks touching it. Immediately lower yourself down slowly, ideally lowering your shoulders and legs to reach the floor at the same time. Focus on controlling your movements, so that the muscles will work as they should. Rest for a couple of seconds, take another deep breath, and repeat. Complete 15 reps, rest for 1 minute, then complete a second set.

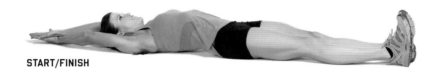

START/FINISH

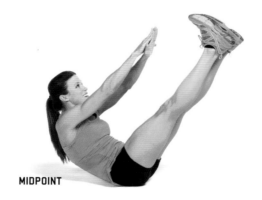

MIDPOINT

Modified Sit-up

Lie on your back with your knees bent and your feet flat on the floor. Raise a leg at least a foot off the floor. Anchor the other leg by either putting your foot under an object or having someone hold it down. Once you get stronger, you will be able to do this without anchoring your foot (see start). Cross your arms over your chest or put your hands on the sides of your head, but don't lock your hands behind your head or support your head with your hands (to avoid pulling on your head, which can cause neck injury).

Take a deep breath and then exhale while rolling your head and shoulders off the ground toward your knees. When your shoulders leave the floor, contract your abs and begin pulling with your hip flexors to bring your back all the way off the floor (see midpoint). Keep moving up as far as you can or until you can touch an elbow to your bent knee, then slowly lower yourself back to the floor. Don't jerk up off the floor when your abs get tired, because this will cause your back muscles to contract and could result in injury. Complete 10 reps on one side, then do another 10 reps on the other side. Rest for 1 minute and complete a second set.

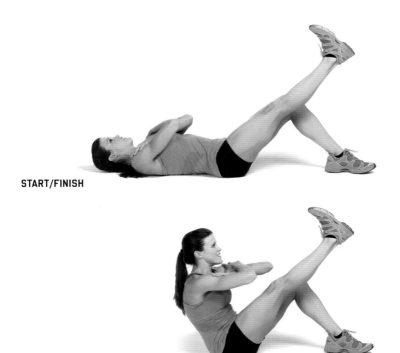

START/FINISH

MIDPOINT

Stability Ball Bridge

Lie on your back with your knees bent and your feet flat against the top of a stability ball. Place your arms at your sides with your palms flat on the floor (see start). (When you get really good at this exercise, put your arms across your chest.)

Push on the ball with your feet to lift your hips up into the air until your body is in a straight line from your knees to your shoulders (see midpoint). Hold this position as long as you can for up to 1 minute, then relax back to the floor. Rest for 15 seconds and repeat three more times. If you want to make this exercise more difficult, hold one foot up in the air, and with the other foot in the middle of the ball, push up into the bridge position (see variation).

CAUTION: If you feel any pain in your neck or cramping in your hamstrings at any point, stop immediately and rest. Pain in your neck or back should be described to your doctor before you continue.

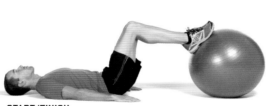

START/FINISH

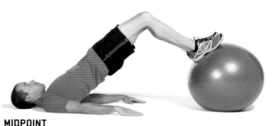

MIDPOINT

VARIATION

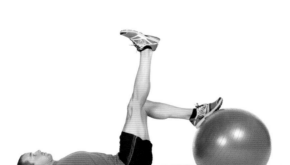

START/FINISH

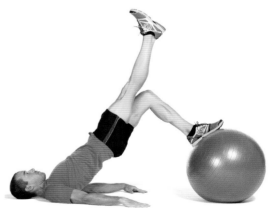

MIDPOINT

Moguls

Lie facedown on your stability ball. Place your hands on the floor right under your shoulders and straighten your arms. Keep your knees and feet together and hold your legs straight out. Slowly walk out on your hands until the ball is under your hips (see start). Hold yourself in this position and keep the ball from moving side to side.

Using your arms to hold your upper body in place, bring your knees up toward your chest while rotating your hips so that your legs move out to your right side and your left leg is the only part of you touching the ball (see midpoint). Straighten back out to the starting position by rolling your legs back under you and straightening them at the same time. Repeat this movement to the left side, bringing your knees up toward your chest and rotating your hips so that only your right leg is touching the ball. Return to the starting position and continue reps side to side. Keep going until you have finished 20 reps, rest for about 1 minute, and do another set.

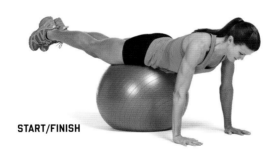

START/FINISH

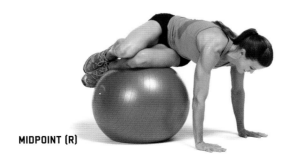

MIDPOINT (R)

Diagonal Wood Chop

Loop your resistance tubing through your door anchor or over a pole above your head. Hold one handle in each hand. Facing the anchor, hold your hands overhead and step back until all the slack is out of the tubing (see start). Stand with your feet shoulder width apart, knees and hips slightly bent.

With a quick downward movement, keeping your arms straight, bring your hands down toward the floor outside your left foot (see midpoint). Bend your knees and hips so that you finish the chop about a foot above the floor. Quickly allow the tubing to pull you back to the start position, and do another rep down toward the floor outside your right foot, then go back to the start position. Continue alternating left and right diagonal chops until you complete 20 reps. Rest about 30 seconds and do another set.

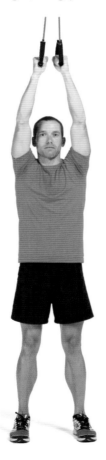

START/FINISH

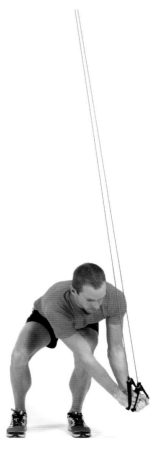

MIDPOINT (L)

Balanced Cross-Pull

GOAL 2 sets of 15 reps on each side

Attach one end of your resistance tubing to your door anchor or around a pole at chest level. Hold the other end in one hand. Stand so that the hand with the tubing is away from the anchor. With your arm held straight across the front of your body, step away from the anchor until there is no slack in the tubing. If the tubing is in your right hand, stand on your left foot; or if the tubing is in your left hand, stand on your right foot (see start).

Keep your arm straight while you slowly pull on the tubing until your arm is pointed out to your side (see finish). This is a full 180 degrees of movement for the arm. Slowly, with control, return to the starting position and complete 10 to 15 reps for this set. Your goal is to keep your body still and balanced on one foot while you pull on the tubing. After a set on one side, switch and do a set on the other side. Complete 2 sets on each side.

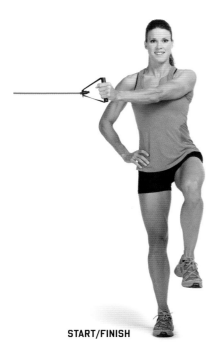

START/FINISH

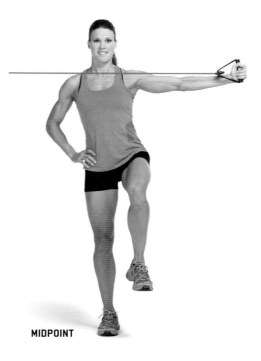

MIDPOINT

Two-Arm Throw

Loop your resistance tubing through your door anchor or under something heavy at ground level. Facing away from the anchor, hold one handle in each hand with an overhand grip, palms facing backward. Hold your hands down at your sides and step forward until you feel the tubing start to pull your arms behind you. Take one more step so that your hands are just behind your buttocks, then stand on one foot (see start).

Keep your arms straight while you quickly pull with both hands until your arms are pointing out in front of you, just above parallel to the floor (see midpoint). Instead of holding that position, let the tubing pull you back to the starting position, and immediately begin another rep. Repeat for 10 to 15 reps, then switch your standing leg and do a set on the other side. Complete 2 to 4 sets, resting 15 to 20 seconds between each set.

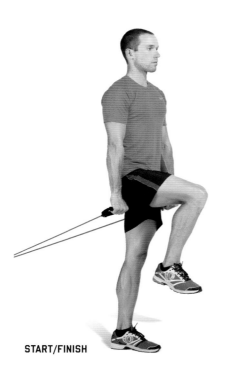

START/FINISH

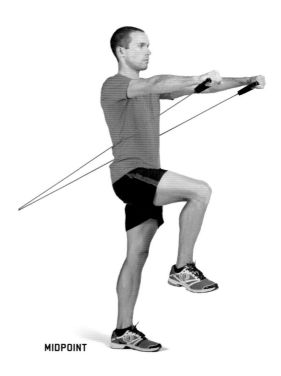

MIDPOINT

Stump Throw

Hold a medicine ball with both hands. Choose a size and weight of ball that is appropriate for your level of training and the intensity you want to achieve. Stand with your feet slightly more than shoulder width apart. Make sure that one foot is not behind the other; they should be even—as if you're standing on a line. Hold the ball down in front of you, arms straight. Squat down until the ball just touches the floor (see start).

Quickly stand up and, at the same time, swing the ball up and out in an arc in front of you; always keeping your arms straight. As the ball is coming up, angle it to one side a bit so that at the top of the swing, when the ball is all the way above you, it is traveling over one shoulder (see midpoint). Slow the ball down as it passes over your shoulder at the top of the swing, and pull the ball back down in the same arc, keeping your arms straight. Bring the ball all the way back to the starting point, letting your hips and knees bend to get back to the squatting position. Immediately change directions and begin another rep, but to the other shoulder. Repeat stump throws over the left and right shoulders until you have completed 20 reps. Rest 15 to 20 seconds, then complete another set.

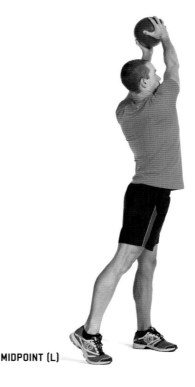

MIDPOINT (L)

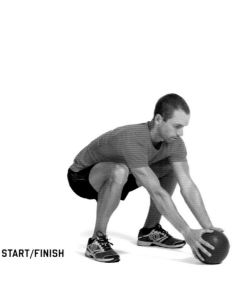

START/FINISH

Standing Russian Twist

GOAL 3 sets of 20 reps

Stand with your feet slightly wider than shoulder width apart. Bend the knees and hips just a little bit so you are not standing up perfectly straight. (Bending the knees and hips allows the legs to absorb some of the rotation, keeping your back from doing too much twisting.) Hold a medicine ball straight out in front of you, with one hand on each side (see start). Use the appropriate size and weight of medicine ball for your ability and the intensity you want to create.

Keep your feet in place. Quickly rotate your body to the left as far as you can (see midpoint). When you get as much twist as you can out of your trunk, quickly rotate all the way around to the right as far as you can. Repeat rotations to the left and right as fast as you can with proper form. Keep the ball out in front of you at shoulder height. If the ball starts to sag, stop and rest, or use a lighter ball. Do 16 to 20 reps, rest 1 minute, and repeat for a total of 3 sets.

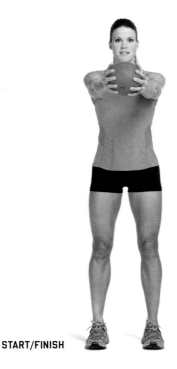

START/FINISH

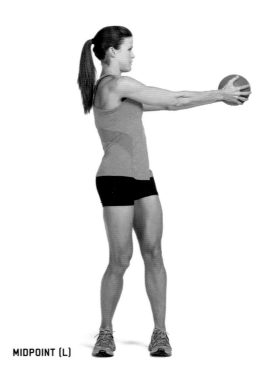

MIDPOINT (L)

Lunging Russian Twist

GOAL 2 sets of 30 reps on each side

Stand with your feet a few inches apart and hold a medicine ball straight out in front of you, with one hand on each side. Use the appropriate size and weight of ball for your ability and the intensity you want to create (see start).

Take a giant step forward with your right foot, like you are stepping over a large puddle of water, allowing your right knee to bend and your left knee to drop toward the ground, but do not allow the left knee to touch the ground. With your right foot out in front, rotate your torso right while keeping your hips facing forward (see finish). Make your rotation quick and powerful—almost as if you were going to throw the ball—moving as far as you can in that direction and quickly moving back to face forward. Keep the ball straight out in front of you as much as you can. Step forward with the left foot and rotate in the other direction (left). Keep stepping until you have completed 30 steps (15 on each side). Rest for 1 minute and do another set.

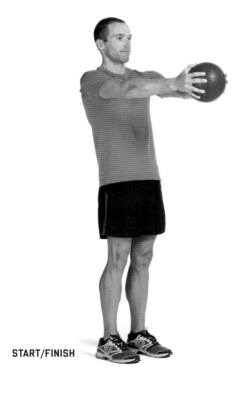

START/FINISH

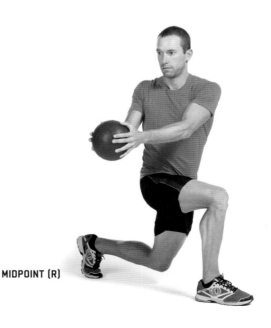

MIDPOINT (R)

Lying Russian Twist

Lie on your back on an exercise mat or a padded surface. Bend your knees and keep your feet flat on the floor, about a foot from your buttocks. Hold a medicine ball in both hands directly above your head and shoulders. Use a ball of the appropriate size and weight for your ability and the intensity you want to create. Keep your arms straight and perform a crunch, lifting your head and shoulders off the floor—then hold that position (see start).

Rotate your body to one side until you can almost touch the ball to the floor next to you. You may have to crunch up a little farther in the starting position in order to keep your shoulders off the floor when you rotate (see midpoint). Rotate back to the starting position and on over to the other side, reaching the ball toward the floor next to you again. Continue rotating left and right for 10 total reps (5 left and 5 right), while keeping your shoulders from touching back down. Relax back to the floor, set the ball down, rest for 30 seconds, then repeat to complete 2 more sets.

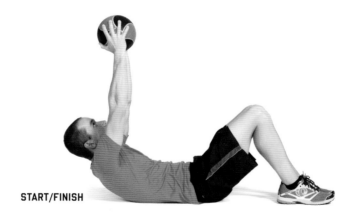

START/FINISH

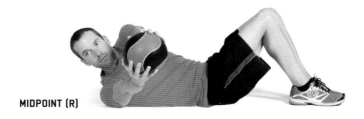

MIDPOINT (R)

Pendulum

Stand with your feet shoulder width apart, knees slightly bent. Hold a medicine ball of the appropriate size and weight for your ability and the intensity you want to create in both hands, one hand on each side of the ball. Hold the ball down in front of you, keeping your arms straight. Bend at the waist as far as you can without bending your knees any more or letting the ball touch the ground. Let your arms and the ball hang down toward the ground in a relaxed position. Keep your back as straight as you can (see start).

Slowly rotate your body to one side, bringing the ball up and out to your left side as far as you can while keeping your back straight (see left midpoint). Let gravity take over and bring you back down to the starting position and on across toward the other side, swinging smoothly like a pendulum. Use your abdominal and lower-back muscles to help swing the ball up and out to your right side as far as you can rotate (see right midpoint). Continue swinging from side to side, each time trying to rotate as far as possible, until you complete 20 total reps (10 on each side). Rest 30 seconds, then repeat to complete 2 more sets.

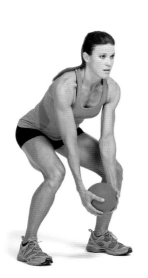

START

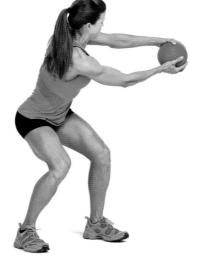

MIDPOINT (L)

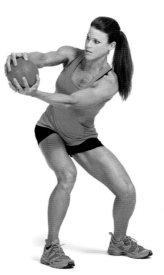

MIDPOINT (R)

CHAPTER 9

Upper-Body Exercises for Swimming

The ability of your arms to pull and push your body through water is a huge part of successful swimming. The pull begins when the hand enters the water and you "pull" it toward your chest. The push occurs at the point where your hand passes your shoulder and starts moving toward your hip. The final phase, recovery, comes after the push, when you return your arm to the starting position.

Upper-body strength training for swimming focuses on the deltoid muscles of the shoulder, which work throughout the stroke movement; the latissimus dorsi (lats) and biceps for the pull phase; the triceps and pectoralis muscles (pecs) for the push phase, then deltoids and triceps for the recovery phase. Unfortunately, there aren't any exercise machines that mimic swimming strokes. The good news is that with a little creativity, you can target the individual muscles used during any stroke, and by combining several exercises, you can work all the upper-body muscles involved in swimming. Some of these exercises focus on the stroke itself; others focus on the recovery phase.

For the exercises that use resistance tubing, the number of repetitions is provided. Choose the proper number of sets and amount of rest for your goal.

One-Arm Throw

MUSCLE FOCUS lats, delts

The one-arm throw focuses on the front portion of your deltoids and on your lats, in a motion that simulates how your upper arm pulls you through the water.

Loop your resistance tubing through a door anchor at the top of a door or around a pole above your head. Hold one handle in one hand, or for more resistance, hold both handles in one hand. Facing away from the anchor, hold your arm over your head and step forward until there is no slack in the tubing and it is just starting to pull you backward. Balance on the leg on the same side as the arm holding the tubing (see start).

Keeping your body upright and still and your arm perfectly straight, quickly pull down on the tubing until your arm is pointing out in front of you (see midpoint), then quickly return it to the starting point. You should be moving with some speed, but don't let the tubing bounce back and forth; always be in control of it. Repeat 10 to 15 times on that side, then switch sides to complete your set.

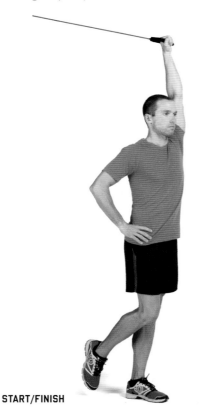

START/FINISH

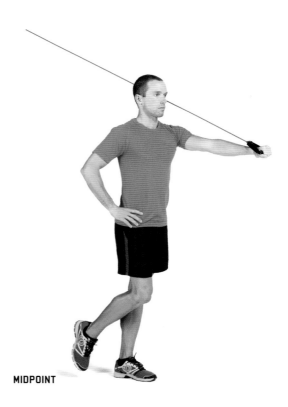

MIDPOINT

Slam Dunk

The slam dunk is all about creating powerful strokes and moving your arms from over your head through a full range of motion down to your side. You won't use both arms at the same time to pull during swimming, but using them together now allows you to get more out of the exercise than if you were to use just one arm.

Stand with your feet about shoulder width apart. Hold a 10- to 15-pound medicine ball in both hands over your head as high as you can reach (see start). Keep a firm grasp on both sides of the ball. With lots of power and speed, quickly throw the ball down toward the floor directly in front of you. Release the ball once it gets to about hip level, before you start bending at the hips (see midpoint). If the ball you are using bounces, it should bounce right back up into your hands. Catch it and let the momentum carry you back to the start position. If the ball doesn't bounce, quickly bend down, pick it up, and lift it back to the start position. When you get the ball back over your head, slam it down again. Repeat slam dunks for 10 to 15 reps per set.

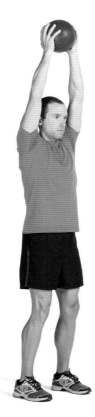

START/FINISH

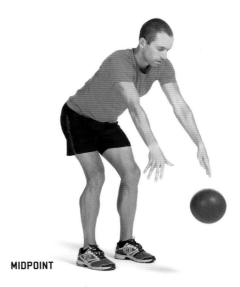

MIDPOINT

Bridging Pullover

MUSCLE FOCUS delts, lats, pecs

The bridging pullover focuses on a powerful pull, and using a stability ball gives the added effect of working with an unstable torso. This exercise will help you learn to pull stronger while keeping your body from moving around too much.

Loop your resistance tubing through your door anchor or around a pole at hip level. Hold one handle in each hand. If this is too much resistance, anchor one end of the tubing and hold the other end in both hands. Sit on your stability ball facing away from the anchor. Holding your arms over your head, lie back on the ball, letting it roll up your back until your shoulders are positioned on top of the ball. Your arms should now be pointing back behind you toward the tubing anchor (see start). Hold

your hips up in the bridge position so that your knees, hips, and shoulders are in a straight line and your back is straight. If there is any slack in the tubing, sit up and move farther away from the anchor.

Keeping your body in the bridging position, pull the tubing up over your head (see midpoint) and then down, until your arms are pointing out in front of you (see finish). Keep your arms completely straight during the entire pull. If you need to raise your head to see where you are pointing, that's fine. Slowly return to the start position while staying in control of the tubing; don't let it pull you back too fast. As you get better at this exercise, you will be able to do it faster and with more power. Do 10 to 15 reps per set.

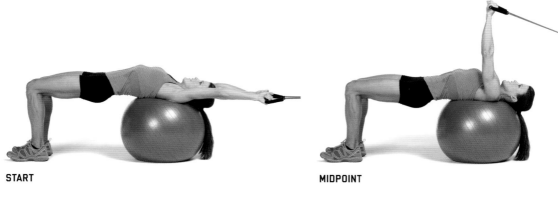

START   MIDPOINT

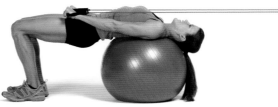

FINISH

Tubing Stroke

MUSCLE FOCUS biceps, delts, lats, pecs, triceps

The tubing stroke is a complete pull-and-push maneuver, exactly what you do while swimming. Everyone has a slightly different stroke style, and this exercise allows you to mimic your own style, with the resistance tubing trying to pull your arm back over your head.

Loop your resistance tubing through a door anchor at the top of the door or around a pole above your head. Kneel on the floor, facing the tubing anchor. Hold one end of the tubing in each hand and lift your arms above your head (see start). There should be no slack in the tubing at the start position; to get rid of slack, shorten the tubing by either loop-

ing it through the anchor again or wrapping it around your hands.

Using one hand at a time, pull the tubing down with your normal stroke movement (see midpoint); once it passes the level of your elbow, push it all the way down to finish the stroke (see finish). Concentrate on moving in your normal stroke pattern, not just on getting your hand down. Let your arm return to the starting position, controlling the movement; don't let the tubing yank your arm back up. Now complete a stroke on the other side. Alternate left and right arms until you have completed 20 to 30 total strokes per set.

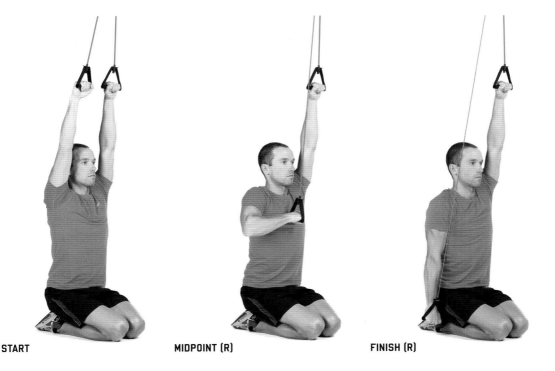

START　　　　　　　**MIDPOINT (R)**　　　　　　　**FINISH (R)**

Dumbbell Shoulder Press

MUSCLE FOCUS delts, triceps

The dumbbell shoulder press is designed to help you straighten out your arm completely prior to beginning a stroke. In the water you won't have as much resistance as the dumbbells provide, so actual swimming will be much easier than this exercise.

Sit on top of your stability ball with your feet spread apart on the floor, slightly wider than shoulder width. Sit up as straight as you can during the entire exercise. Hold a dumbbell in each hand at shoulder level, either in front of or just to the sides of your shoulders (see start), whichever is more comfortable for you. Your palms should be facing away from you.

Push both dumbbells over your head at the same time until your arms are completely straight. As you press them up, think about trying to move them in a straight line from your shoulders to directly over your head. Don't let them sway forward or backward, as this wastes energy and means you aren't in control of them. The dumbbells will naturally move closer together as you push up, and they can touch at the very top of the press (see midpoint). Slowly lower the dumbbells back to the starting position. If this exercise is difficult, have a spotter stand behind you to make sure you don't drop a dumbbell.

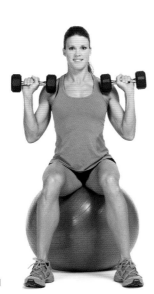

START/FINISH

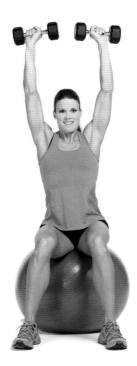

MIDPOINT

Tubing Kickback

The tubing kickback also mimics the final push of your stroke, but with just one hand at a time.

Attach one end of your resistance tubing to your door anchor or loop it around a pole at chest level and hold the other end of the tubing in one hand. Place the free hand on your thigh. Bend forward slightly at the hips, keeping your back straight. Bend the arm holding the tubing, lifting your elbow up until your upper arm is parallel to the floor, or as close to parallel as possible; your shoulder and elbow should be at the same height (see start). Keep your hand as close to your shoulder as possible. Now back up until there is some stretch and resistance in the tubing.

Concentrate on keeping your body, elbow, and shoulder still as you straighten out your arm behind you, pulling the tubing out. Pull on the tubing until your arm is completely straight and pointing behind you (see midpoint). Slowly let your elbow bend again, bringing your hand back to your shoulder. Don't let the tubing control the movement and snap back too quickly. Do 10 to 15 reps, then switch sides to complete a set.

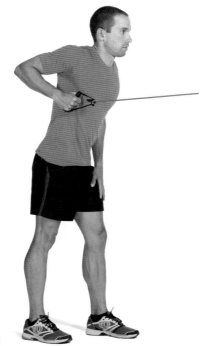

START/FINISH

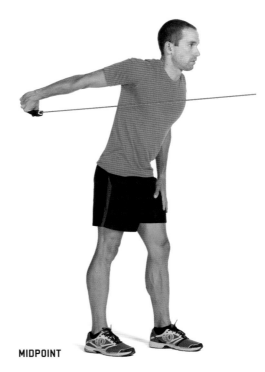

MIDPOINT

Dumbbell Curl

MUSCLE FOCUS biceps

If you watch how your arm moves during the initial pull of your stroke, you will notice that the elbow has to bend to keep your hand close to your body. The biceps make this possible and determine how strong your pull will be.

Hold a dumbbell in each hand using an underhand grip (palms facing forward). Stand with your feet shoulder width apart and your knees slightly bent, letting the dumbbells rest against the outside of your thighs (see start). Your arms should be completely straight.

To keep from swaying, perform the dumbbell curl one arm at a time, alternating arms. Slowly bend your elbow and bring the dumbbell up to shoulder height (see midpoint). When curling, keep your elbows at your side so the only part of your body that is moving is your forearm and hand. Slowly lower the dumbbell until your arm is completely straight again. Alternate left and right curls until your set is complete.

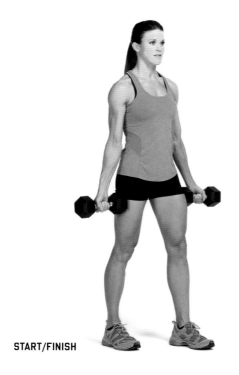

START/FINISH

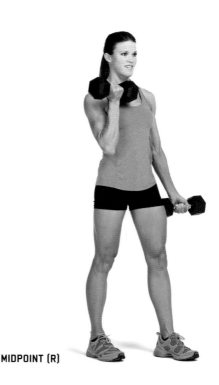

MIDPOINT (R)

Triceps Push-down

The triceps push-down concentrates on the last half of your stroke, the push. The relatively small triceps muscles have to provide the last push to propel you through the water, so training them is essential.

Attach a straight or V-shaped handle to a high-pulley cable machine, which supports the best technique for this exercise. Face the machine and grasp the handle with an overhand grip (palms facing down), making sure your hands are evenly spaced from the middle to prevent tilting. Bend your elbows, keeping them close to your sides. Your hands should come as close to your shoulders as possible while holding your elbows in the start position (see start). Stand as close to the cable as possible. If you find that you have to push the handles away from your body during the exercise, take a small step back so you can push the cable down in a straight line.

Keeping your elbows at your sides, push down on the handle until both arms are completely straight (see midpoint). Slowly let your elbows bend to bring the handle back to the start position. Throughout the entire movement, your elbows should remain at your sides; only your forearms and hands should be moving. Repeat the motion until your set is complete.

If you want a bigger challenge, do this exercise one arm at a time using a single-hand attachment.

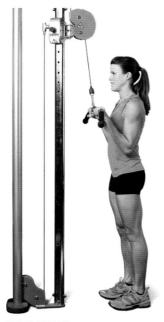

START/FINISH

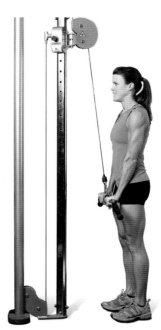

MIDPOINT

Dumbbell Fly

The dumbbell fly is the only exercise that isolates the pecs for movement, with the delts providing stability for the arms, thus letting you train the pecs more than on any other exercise. It really helps the recovery phase of your stroke.

Lie on your back on a stability ball so the ball is underneath your shoulder blades and your legs are bent at a 90-degree angle in front of you. Lift your pelvis up toward the ceiling to create a straight-line bridge from your shoulders to your knees, and hold it steady. Your feet can be placed as close together as is comfortable. The wider your feet are spaced, the easier the exercise is. Hold a dumbbell in each hand and extend your arms upward, palms facing each other, positioning the dumbbells over your chest and shoulders—never over your head. Begin with the dumbbells touching, and to prevent any elbow strain, bend your elbows slightly. Keep your arms "locked" in this position so your elbows don't bend farther when you perform the exercise (see start).

Inhale deeply, and slowly lower the dumbbells to your sides, as if you were getting ready to hug a very big tree. Lower the dumbbells until they are slightly higher than your shoulders (see midpoint and alternate view). Avoid lowering below shoulder level, as this can cause elbow hyperextension and potential injury. Exhale as you bring the dumbbells back up to the starting point over your chest. Keep the slight bend in your arms so the movement doesn't become a dumbbell press. Repeat the motion until your set is complete.

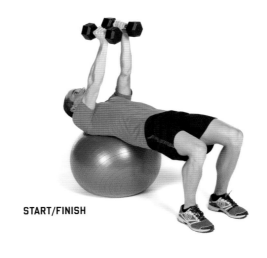

START/FINISH

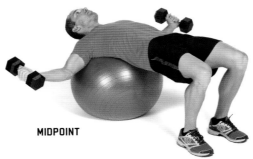

MIDPOINT

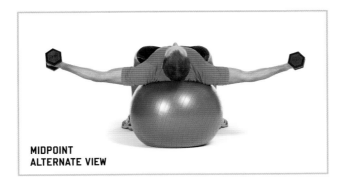

MIDPOINT
ALTERNATE VIEW

Dip

The dip is one of the most difficult but useful exercises in this book. It combines extension of the elbow from the triceps with flexion of the shoulder from the deltoids to double the force of your push.

Use a dip stand specially made for doing this exercise. A dip stand is sometimes combined with a knee raise stand or a pull-up stand. The arms of the stand usually are not adjustable, but if they are, adjust them so that they are just wider than your hips. Use the steps provided to get up to the start position. Place a hand on each of the dip stand arms, palms facing toward your body. It's best to grasp the bar with your thumb on one side and your fingers on the other so your hand can't slip off during the exercise. Press yourself up until your arms are completely straight and are holding your body up, unsupported by the legs. Cross your feet at your ankles and bend your knees so you don't touch the steps or the floor at the midpoint of this exercise (see start).

Slowly bend your elbows and lower yourself toward the floor until your shoulders and elbows are at the same level and your upper arms are parallel to the floor (see midpoint). Once you have reached this position, push with both hands to straighten your arms until your elbows are perfectly straight again and you are back at the starting position.

If you don't have a dip stand or find this exercise too difficult, you can use a flat bench and do a variation of the dip called the seated dip. Place your hands on the edge of the bench, palms facing away from you and arms straightened, and slide your legs straight out in front of you until you are in a bridge position (see variation start). Slowly lower your hips toward the floor, until your shoulders and elbows are at the same height and your upper arms are parallel to the floor (see variation midpoint). (If you end up sitting on the floor, find a taller bench.) Push up to return to the starting position, with arms straightened. Complete 3 sets of 10 reps

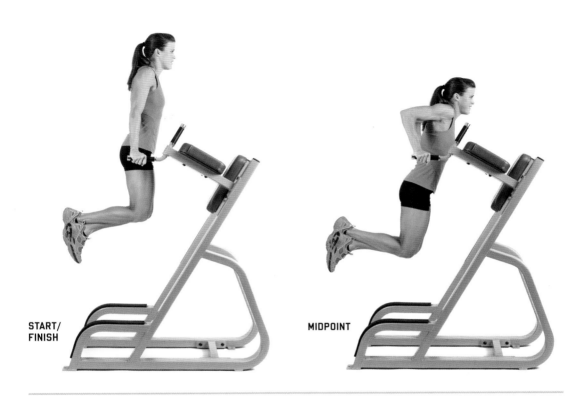

START/
FINISH

MIDPOINT

VARIATION

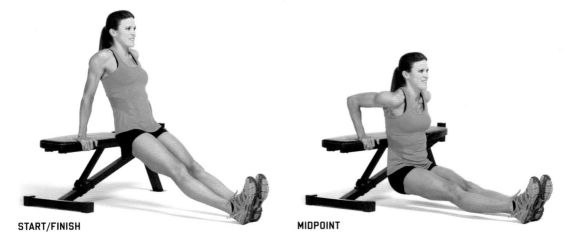

START/FINISH

MIDPOINT

Dumbbell Lateral Raise

MUSCLE FOCUS delts

The dumbbell lateral raise focuses on the middle portion of the deltoids, which is mainly responsible for lifting your arm out to the side—a major movement in the recovery phase of the stroke.

Stand with your feet apart, one foot slightly behind the other for balance. Hold a dumbbell in each hand against the outside of your thighs, palms facing your legs (see start). Keeping your arms straight or just slightly bent at the elbow, lift both arms out to your sides until the dumbbells are at shoulder height (see midpoint). Slowly lower them back to your sides. Do not let them drop too quickly; the exercise will be half as effective if you neglect to work your muscles on the way down, too.

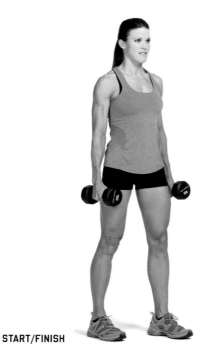

START/FINISH

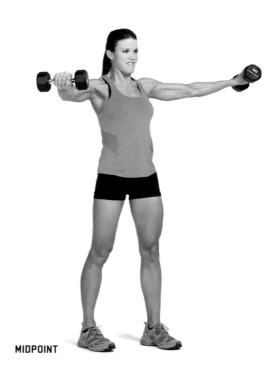

MIDPOINT

Dumbbell Angled Raise

MUSCLE FOCUS delts

This exercise targets the rear portion of the deltoids, which is typically the weakest part because it is only responsible for pulling your arm down and back—a movement that the lats assist with as well. Training with this exercise helps keep the deltoid muscles in balance and lends some assistance to the lats.

Stand with your feet shoulder width apart, one foot slightly in front of the other for balance. Hold a dumbbell in each hand. For this exercise, you will probably use a lighter weight than you would for a front or lateral dumbbell raise because the back portion of the shoulder is typically not as strong. Turn your hands so that your thumbs are pointing toward your legs (see start). This is an odd way to hold a dumbbell, but you will get used to it.

Keep your thumb pointed toward the floor as you lift one dumbbell to shoulder level (see midpoint). When you lift the dumbbell, don't move your arm straight out in front of you or straight out to your side, but halfway in between, diagonal to your body. Slowly return the dumbbell down to your leg and repeat with the other arm. Alternate arms to complete the set.

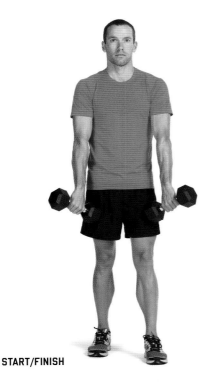

START/FINISH

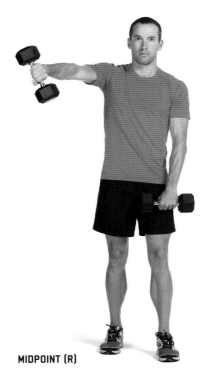

MIDPOINT (R)

CHAPTER 10

Lower-Body Exercises for Swimming

Although the upper body may be the powerhouse during swimming, the lower body provides a good deal of propulsion and stability in the water. During your swim training you probably do drills that focus on just the upper or the lower body, which is why you need to do strength training that focuses on each part as well. The lower body, which includes your hips, thighs, and calves, doesn't provide a lot of buoyancy, so you have to keep it moving during the swim to prevent dragging your legs along at the expense of your arms. Strength training for the lower body won't provide a huge increase in your swimming speed or performance, but you will see its effects when you transition to the bike and run, where your legs are most important.

Lower-body strength training for swimming focuses on the glute muscles (gluteus maximus and medius), which extend your hip to the back and side; the hamstrings, which help with hip extension; the adductor group, which is responsible for keeping your legs close together; the quadriceps, which are strong knee extensors and hip flexors; and the calves, which point the feet and toes.

Cable Lateral Lift

The cable lateral lift focuses on the often-ignored smaller glute muscle, the gluteus medius. This muscle is responsible for lifting your leg out to your side and for stabilizing the larger gluteus maximus during hip extension. Training this muscle will help keep your legs from flailing out to the sides and will allow you to concentrate on extending your hip with each kick.

Attach the ankle strap of a low-pulley machine to one leg. Stand so that the leg you are going to work is farthest away from the machine and the cable crosses in front of you.

Hold on to the machine with one hand and place the other hand on your hip (see start).

Keep your body as straight as possible while you lift your leg directly out to the side as high as you can (see midpoint). Concentrate on moving your leg to the side and not forward or backward. If you start to lean your upper body toward the machine, that's as high as you can go; leaning doesn't work the glute muscles. Slowly bring your leg back down and repeat until your reps are complete, then switch sides and do the same number of reps to complete your set.

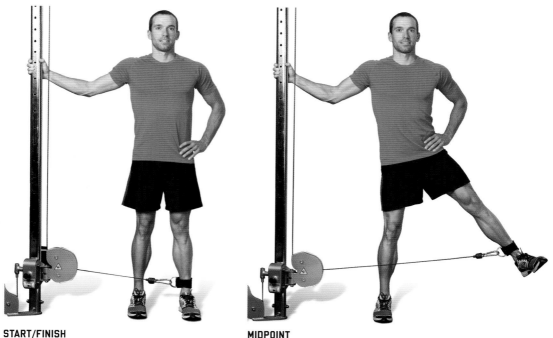

START/FINISH   **MIDPOINT**

Inclined Superman

MUSCLE FOCUS gluteus maximus, hamstrings

The inclined superman locks your knees straight while you use your glutes and hamstrings to extend your hips. By keeping your knees locked, you are able to make the hamstrings work at the hip, effectively increasing the force of hip extension during your kick.

Facing away from a wall, lie facedown over your stability ball. Anchor your feet by setting your toes on the floor and your heels against the wall. Keep your legs straight. Position the ball so that the top is at your waist and your head is lower than your hips. Hold your arms straight out over your head, touching the floor (see start).

Take a deep breath, then exhale as you lift your upper body off the ball as high as you can (see midpoint). Your upper legs and hips will stay on the ball. Really focus on squeezing your glutes, and if you feel this in your lower back, that's normal; those muscles are supporting your upper body. Slowly relax back to the start position, then repeat for 10 to 15 times per set. If you need more resistance, hold a medicine ball in your hands.

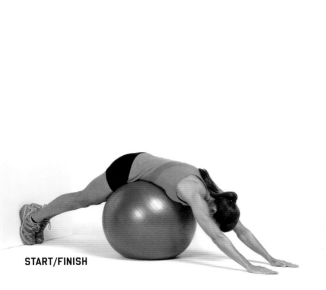

START/FINISH

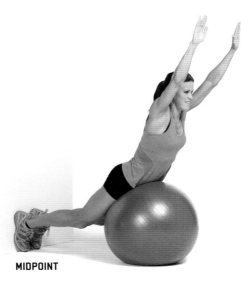

MIDPOINT

Leg Extension

This exercise concentrates on the force that you produce while extending your knees, which is critical for a solid kick. The leg extension machine has a bad rap as an exercise that will hurt your knees. There is minimal evidence for this, and it usually involves people who have had a previous knee injury. If your knees hurt, don't do this exercise, but if they are healthy, performing it correctly should not cause any damage.

Sit down on the leg extension machine and line up your knees with the machine's pivot point. On some machines, this requires adjusting the seat back. The pivot point is usually evident (or can be found on the machine's instruction card) and is usually at the edge of the seat. If your knees are too far forward, there will be a lot of strain on them at the start of the exercise. Place your feet behind

the footpad and adjust it so the pad rests just above your feet on your shins (see start). (Some machines adjust themselves, so you may not have to do this.) If you can adjust how far under the seat the leg pad is, move it so that you start with your knees bent at about a 90-degree angle. Too tight an angle at the start can cause some knee pain, especially if you have had a knee injury.

Holding onto the handles or sides of the seat, straighten out your legs as far as possible. The goal is to get your legs completely extended (see midpoint). Slowly lower your legs back down to a point just before the weight stack comes to a rest, then repeat until your set is complete.

CAUTION: If your knees hurt at all during this exercise, skip it and use another exercise.

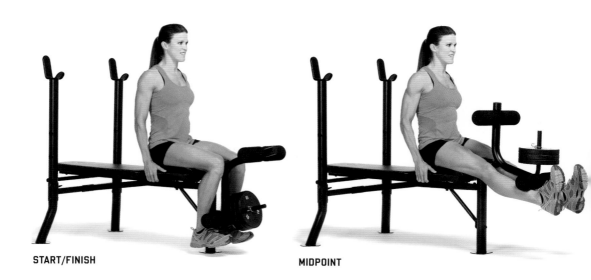

START/FINISH   **MIDPOINT**

Cable Hip Extension

MUSCLE FOCUS gluteus maximus, hamstrings

The cable hip extension allows you to work through the same range of motion that the hip uses during swimming. You can alter the range of motion you use here to fit you best.

Attach the ankle strap of a low-pulley machine to one leg. Stand facing the machine and hold on to it with both hands. Step back until your arms are straight and there is just a little pull on the cable. Put all your weight on your support leg and keep your body as upright as possible (see start).

Keeping your leg straight, push it back as far as you can (see midpoint). This is not a large motion, so focus on squeezing your glutes. You may be tempted to lean your body forward to get more range of motion, but this actually decreases the effectiveness of the exercise. Slowly return to the start position, then repeat until your reps are complete. Switch legs and do the same number of reps on the opposite side to complete your set.

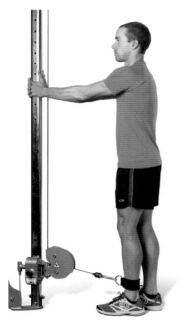

START/FINISH

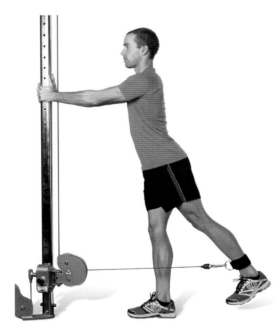

MIDPOINT

Cable Lateral Cross

The adductor muscles used during the cable lateral cross are responsible for helping the gluteus medius stabilize the hip and the gluteus maximus. Performing this exercise will also help with your hip extension force by keeping the leg moving in the correct direction.

Attach the ankle strap of a low-pulley machine to one leg. Stand so that the leg you are going to work is closest to the machine. Place both hands on your hips and step away from the machine until your working leg is being pulled toward it (see start). Put all your weight on the other leg. If you feel off balance, hold on to the machine with one hand.

Pull your extended leg back toward your support leg and then across in front of you as far as possible (see midpoint). As you move, make sure that the only part of you that is moving is your leg. Don't let your shoulders or hips turn toward the machine in an effort to move your leg farther. Slowly return back to the start position, then repeat until your reps are complete. Switch legs and complete the same number of reps on the opposite side to complete your set.

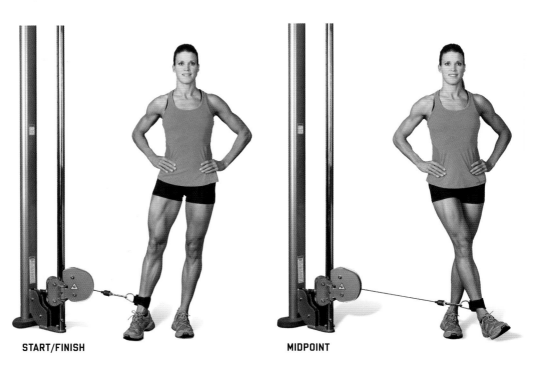

START/FINISH

MIDPOINT

Lying Leg Curl

The lying leg curl mimics the position of swimming better than other leg curl exercises. Though you are not bending your knees that much during swimming, the hamstring muscles cross both the knee and hip joint, so they aid in moving your leg at the hip during the recovery phase of your kick.

Find the pivot point of the lying leg curl machine. Usually it is right at the edge of the padding. Stand at the end of the bench with your knees right against the padding and lie facedown. Your kneecaps should hang off the end of the bench and line up with the machine's pivot point. Lie all the way down and hold on to the handles. (Some machines have pads for your elbows to rest on; others have a flat bench to rest your chest and head on. Either is fine.) Your feet should be underneath the leg pad (see start). Some machines adjust this automatically, but if yours does not, adjust the pad so it is in contact with the backs of your legs, just below your calves (on your Achilles tendon), and is not pushing on your foot.

Bend your knees, pulling the foot pad up as far as you can (see midpoint). The goal is to get the pad all the way to your buttocks. The farther you can curl your legs, the more you benefit from this exercise. Try to keep your hips flat on the pad during the motion. If they start to rise, hold them down by tightening your glutes. Slowly lower the weight back down, then repeat until your set is complete.

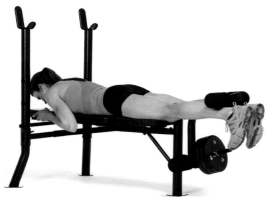

START/FINISH

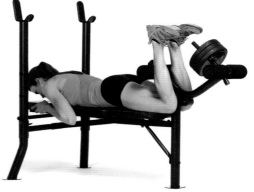

MIDPOINT

Seated Calf Raise

The seated calf raise mainly works the smaller calf muscle, the soleus. This muscle is a very strong endurance-oriented muscle that keeps your feet pointed while swimming.

Sit down on the machine and place your feet on the footplate so that just the balls of your feet are on the plate and your heels are hanging off the back. Slide your knees under the pads and adjust them so they are snug against your knees but not pushing down hard (see start). You can hold on to the hand grips, but make sure not to pull the knee pad up with your hands during the exercise—that job must be done by your calves.

Push on the balls of your feet to raise your heels as high as you can (see midpoint). On the first rep, the bar that supports the machine will move out of the way. Lower your heels as far as you can to get a good stretch. When you can't go down any farther, push back up on the balls of your feet to get back to the highest point you can reach. Repeat, lowering and raising your heels until you have finished all your reps. On the last rep, when you are at the highest point of the exercise, move the support bar back under the machine and lower the bar back down on it.

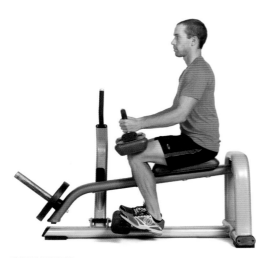

START/FINISH

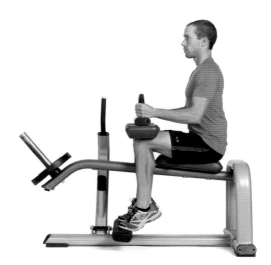

MIDPOINT

Standing Calf Raise

In the standing calf raise you will work both the soleus and the gastrocnemius muscles of the calf. The gastrocnemius provides more power to your kick and helps the soleus.

Stand with your legs together. You can do this exercise standing flat on the floor, but by standing on the edge of a step, curb, aerobics bench, or even a piece of wood, you will get a larger range of motion and better results. If you use a step, stand on the very edge of it so just the balls of your feet are on it and let your heels hang over the edge (see start). Hold on to something in front of you for support.

Let your heels drop as far toward the floor as possible, then push up on the balls of your feet until you can't go any higher (see midpoint). Be sure both legs are pushing evenly; don't let one leg do all the work. Slowly lower your heels back toward the floor and repeat until your set is finished. Complete 3 sets of 20 reps.

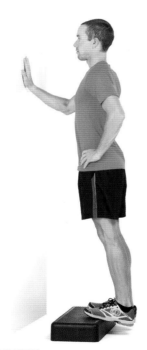

START/FINISH

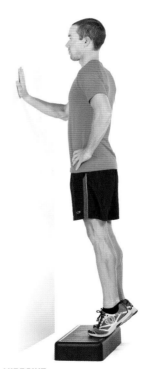

MIDPOINT

Lying Leg Lift

This exercise targets the smaller glute muscle, the gluteus medius, which is responsible for lifting your leg out to the side. While you don't make that particular movement much while swimming, this muscle also assists in stabilizing the hip and assists the other glute muscles. Strengthening it will provide more power to each kick.

Attach an ankle weight to the leg you want to work first. Lie on your side on the floor with that leg on top. Position your bottom arm (the one on the floor) straight out over your head, and rest your head on it. Do not prop yourself up on your elbow. Bend your bottom leg (the one on the floor) so your knee is in front of your body and your foot is behind you. This will provide a solid foundation to keep you upright. Your free hand (the top hand) should rest on your hip or waist. Don't place this hand on the floor, because you will end up pushing against it instead of relying on your glutes for support. Hold your upper leg completely straight, just off the ground (see start), and relax your foot (it doesn't help to point your toe).

Slowly lift your top leg into the air as far as you can (see midpoint). Do not use momentum or thrust your leg up into the air; you should be in complete control and be able to stop moving at any time, so move slowly. Once you have lifted the leg as far as you possibly can, slowly lower it back down toward the floor, stopping just before you make contact. Don't let the lifting leg touch down; keep the resistance throughout the full set. Complete your reps, then move the ankle weight to the other leg and complete a set on that side. Complete 3 sets of 20 reps.

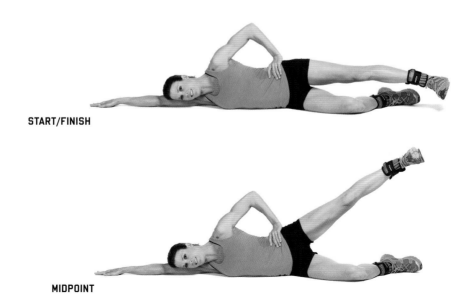

START/FINISH

MIDPOINT

Lateral Lunge

MUSCLE FOCUS glutes, hamstrings, quads

This exercise has a very large eccentric component that targets all of the leg muscles, making them stronger without using much weight. It combines several movements used in swimming (knee and hip extension, hip adduction, plantar flexion) so you get a great all-around leg exercise.

Stand with your feet slightly apart, with your toes pointed slightly out. Hold a pair of dumbbells at shoulder height (see start), but if it's too intense, ditch the dumbbells and place your hands on your hips.

Take a giant step out directly to one side while keeping the opposite foot in place. When your stepping foot lands, put all your weight on that foot and bend your knee. Drop into the lunge until your thigh is parallel to the floor. If you can't bend deep enough to be parallel, just go as far as is comfortable. Your supporting leg should remain straight (see midpoint). Push up out of the lunge to propel yourself back to the starting position. Don't push so hard that you lose your balance, but push hard enough that you don't have to take an additional step or drag your foot back to the starting point. Repeat the lunge to the other side, and alternate reps from side to side until the set is complete.

CAUTION: This exercise can be hard on the knees if you don't take a big enough step or if you bend too deeply. When you drop down into the lunge, don't allow your knee to move laterally past your toes. Also, if your heel lifts off the ground, you didn't step out wide enough. Take a bigger step on your next rep.

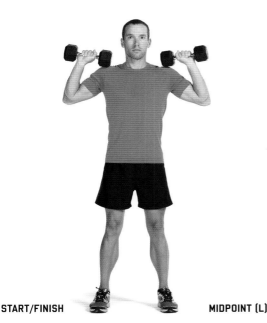

START/FINISH

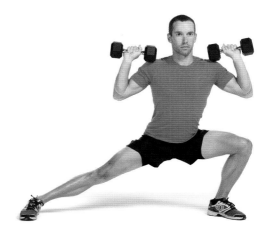

MIDPOINT (L)

Prone Extension

Attach ankle weights to your legs and lie face-down on the floor. You can lie with your chin on your folded arms for more comfort. Place your feet together, with your legs straight and your toes pointed toward the ground (see start).

Keep one leg on the floor while you lift the other leg as high as you can without rolling your body or lifting your hip off the ground (see mid-point). Contract your glutes to hold your leg up for a count of 3 seconds. Then lower your foot back to the floor, but just as it touches, lift it back up again. Don't rest between reps. Switch to the other leg and complete the same number of reps to finish your set. Complete 2 sets of 15 reps.

START/FINISH

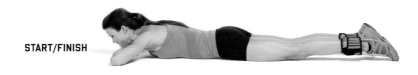

MIDPOINT

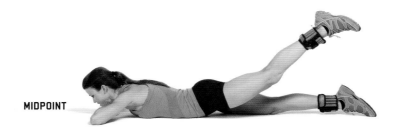

CHAPTER 11

Upper-Body Exercises for Cycling

Many strength training programs for cycling focus on the legs, which makes sense because the legs have been assumed to provide all the propulsion. However, a study of basic biomechanics shows that although the legs do push the pedals and turn the crank, they are only able to do so if the upper body provides a base to push against. Newton's third law of motion states that for every action there is an equal and opposite reaction. In the case of cycling, as you push on the pedals, they push back against you. The only reason the crank turns is that you have a support system at the other end that keeps you from simply standing up each time you push down. Think of how much power you produce, or how hard you can ride, when you are in your normal riding position compared to how hard you can ride when you aren't holding the handlebars at all. The amount of force you can produce always drops when you let go of the handles because your base of support is gone. It does not require a huge amount of strength to provide this support; merely holding the handles is usually enough, until your legs start to fade and the upper body has to work harder.

In addition, your upper body must support the weight of your torso as you lean over the handlebars, whether in a traditional or an aerobar position. Your lower body is supported by the seat, but the bulk of the work required to hold your upper body in position is done by the arms, shoulders, and back. Increasing the performance of these muscles with cycling-specific exercises will decrease your fatigue during cycling and give you more energy during the run.

This chapter focuses on the lower-back muscles (collectively called the erector spinae), upper-back muscles (trapezius, rhomboids), shoulders (deltoids), chest (pectoralis major), triceps, and wrist flexors.

Back Extension

The back extension exercise is the only one that focuses on the erector spinae muscles, which are responsible for keeping your back straight. As these muscles tire, you start to slouch, which puts additional strain on the rest of your body. Keeping your back straight while cycling helps with aerodynamics and to prevent a tight back later, during the run.

Using a 45-degree back extension bench, adjust the height of the thigh pad so that it is just below your waist and allows you to fully bend over without pressing into your stomach. Mount the bench, making sure your heels are set against the heel pads or heel plate that locks your legs so that you don't fall off. Your legs should remain straight during the exercise, but you may turn your toes out to the sides to relieve the pressure on your thighs. Cross your arms over your chest and slowly lower your upper body over the bench by bending at the waist (see start). The goal is to get as far down as you can, so really relax your back and shoulder muscles.

Starting with your lower back, slowly roll yourself up one vertebra at a time, the way a cat arches its back (see midpoint). It will take some practice to activate these small muscles individually. Do not try to hold your back flat or straight. Your shoulders should be the last part of your back that unrolls. Roll up to the point at which your body is in a straight line (see finish)—any further is hyperextension of the spine, which is undesirable. Hold this position briefly and repeat the motion until your set is complete. Do 3 sets of 15 reps.

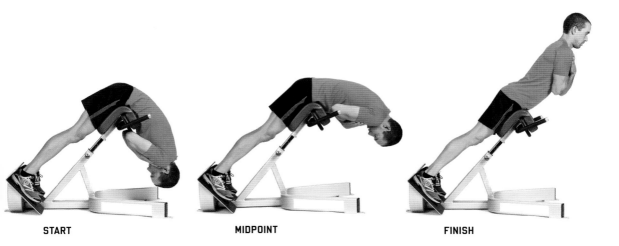

START   **MIDPOINT**   **FINISH**

Protraction

Protraction is a very small movement, but it is very important for keeping your upper back and shoulders in a strong position during your ride. The pecs and front portion of the deltoids work together to pull your shoulders forward, effectively pushing your back into a straight position and keeping your shoulders from tiring.

Attach a resistance tube to an anchor or wrap it around a pole a couple of feet off the floor. Sit on the floor facing away from the anchor, holding one end of the resistance tubing in each hand. Straighten your arms out in front of you and relax your shoulders to let the tubing pull your arms and shoulders back (see start).

Push out on the tubing handles, bringing your shoulders as far forward as possible. Hold the rest of your body still; don't lean forward to move the handles. This exercise only takes about 4 to 6 inches of movement, and it all has to come from the shoulders (see midpoint). Now let your shoulders be pulled back again, fully relax them, and repeat until your set is finished.

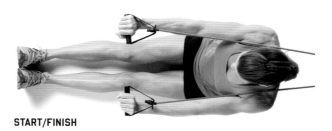

START/FINISH

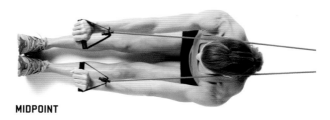

MIDPOINT

Dumbbell Incline Press

MUSCLE FOCUS delts, pecs, triceps

If your bike is set up correctly, your hands will be positioned slightly in front of your shoulders while on top of the handlebars. This exercise builds upper-body stability by replicating the force that you must counter to hold your body in the correct position.

Holding a pair of dumbbells, sit back on an incline exercise bench. If you are using an adjustable bench, set the angle to be about 45 degrees. Position the dumbbells so they are next to your shoulders, palms facing for-ward, with your elbows pointed out to the sides (see start). Press both dumbbells into the air directly over your head until your arms are completely straight (see midpoint). It is important to keep the dumbbells over your head and not let them stray forward or backward—that wastes energy. Slowly lower the dumbbells back to your shoulders and repeat until your set is finished.

NOTE: You may want to use a spotter for this exercise.

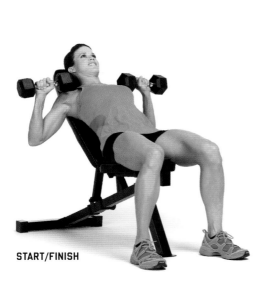

START/FINISH

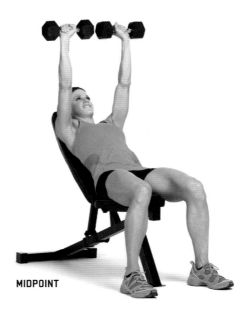

MIDPOINT

Dumbbell Handle Push-up

MUSCLE FOCUS delts, pecs, triceps

The dumbbell handle push-up takes a regular push-up and gives it greater range of motion so that the shoulders, chest, and triceps work more. Sometimes during a ride, especially while facing a strong headwind, you may drop your body lower over the handlebars to create a more aerodynamic position. This exercise helps you hold that position and then push back up out of it when you need to.

Place a pair of dumbbells on the floor in front of you. Get down on your hands and knees and grab the dumbbell handles, positioning them so they are lined up horizontally (perpendicular to the length of your body) and your hands are positioned on the weights directly under your shoulders. Your palms will be facing your knees. The farther apart your hands are, the less effective and sport-specific this exercise becomes. Stretch out your legs behind you and put your feet next to each other or no more than a couple of inches apart. Your toes should be the only part of your body touching the ground. Keep your body rigid and maintain a straight line with your shoulders, hips, and feet (see start). Don't let your hips sag, and don't stick your buttocks up in the air; your entire body must move together and be straight as a board.

Slowly lower yourself toward the floor by bending your arms until either your chest comes in contact with the floor or your shoulders are lower than your elbows (see midpoint). Don't go down so far that you are lying on the floor; just get close and then push yourself back to the start position. It helps to breathe in as you lower yourself and breathe out as you push back up.

If you have trouble completing a push-up in this position, you can do a modified push-up on your knees rather than your toes (see variation start). In this position, you'll keep your body rigid with shoulders, hips, and knees aligned in the modified position (see variation midpoint).

This is a body-weight-only exercise. Do not attempt to make it more difficult by placing weights on your back. If you want to make it harder, wear a proper weighted vest or do more reps.

The push-up, and its variations, is one of the most basic body-weight exercises; yet it is often a difficult exercise for many athletes. Set a goal of completing 3 sets of 20 reps, and if you can't get there right away, keep working on it until you can. As you gain muscular endurance in this exercise, decrease the rest between sets until you are doing one solid set of 60 reps.

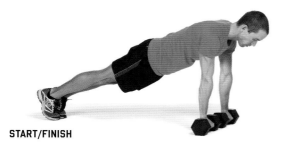

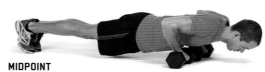

START/FINISH

MIDPOINT

VARIATION

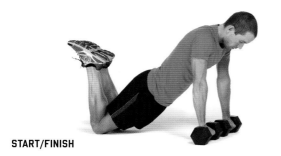

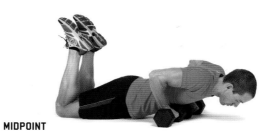

START/FINISH

MIDPOINT

Shoulder Dip

MUSCLE FOCUS rhomboids, trapezius

The shoulder dip gets right to the muscles of your upper back, which tire easily if they aren't trained. The trapezius and rhomboids keep your shoulders in a stable position during your ride, and this exercise forces them to do all the work.

Use a dip stand specially made for doing dips. Use the steps provided to get up to the start position. Place a hand on each of the dip stand arms, palms facing each other. It is best to grasp the bar with your thumb on one side and your fingers on the other so that your hand can't slip off. Press yourself up until your arms are completely straight and step off the stand.

Now keep your arms straight and let your body sag between your shoulders (see start). This will cause your shoulders to move up toward your ears. Keeping the rest of your body and your arms motionless, push down on your hands and raise your entire body up a few inches. Your shoulders should move down as your head moves up (see midpoint). This exercise only takes about 3 to 4 inches of movement, so do it slowly and concentrate on pushing your chest out and pulling your shoulder blades back. Once at the top of the movement, lower yourself back to the start position and finish your reps. Complete 3 sets of 12 reps.

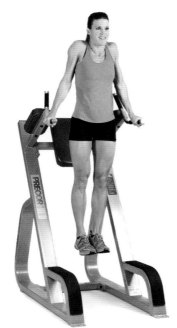

START/FINISH

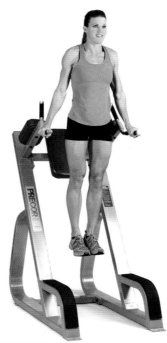

MIDPOINT

Dumbbell Front Raise

MUSCLE FOCUS delts

The front raise is designed to make sure your shoulders are strong enough to support your upper body while on your bike. When you are bent over the handlebars on the bike, your shoulders have to bear the brunt of your upper-body weight and maintain proper position.

Stand with your feet shoulder width apart, one foot staggered in front of the other for stability. Hold a dumbbell in each hand, with your palms facing your legs (see start). Slowly lift one dumbbell straight out in front of you until it is at shoulder height (see midpoint). Your arm should remain as straight as possible throughout the movement. Slowly lower the dumbbell back to your leg, then repeat with the other arm, alternating arms until you have completed all your reps.

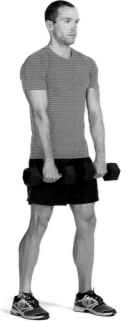

START/FINISH

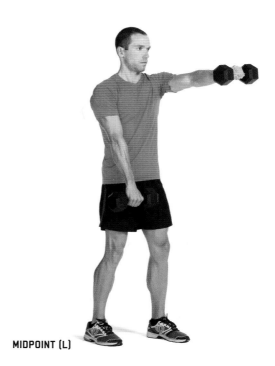

MIDPOINT (L)

Barbell Wrist Curl

MUSCLE FOCUS wrist flexors

The wrist flexors, located mainly in the fore-arms, are often overlooked in training for cycling, which is unfortunate because the first muscles that have to work to hold you in position on the bike are in your hands and fore-arms. If you have ever experienced numbness in your hands during a long ride, this exercise will help by training the wrist to stay in a stronger position that allows better blood flow.

Holding a barbell with both hands, with palms facing away from you in an underhand grip, sit on the end of an exercise bench or a chair. Place your feet about a foot apart and lay the tops of your forearms on your thighs so that only your hands hang off past your knees. Adjust your hands so that they are as far apart as your knees. Let your wrists relax down toward the ground while keeping a firm grip on the barbell (see start).

Curl your wrists up as far as you can, pulling with both hands at the same time. Keep your forearms firmly planted on your thighs during the movement (see midpoint). Let your wrists return to the start position and repeat until your reps are complete.

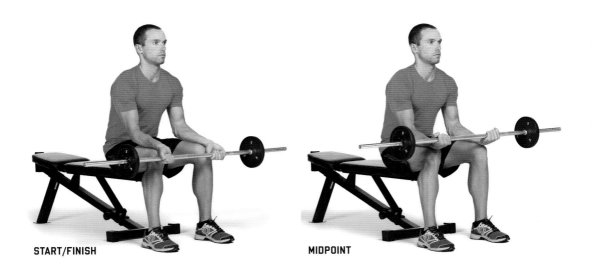

START/FINISH   MIDPOINT

Barbell Front Raise

The barbell front raise targets the shoulder muscles that stabilize the arms while riding, and it mimics the position your arms are in while riding.

Stand with your feet shoulder width apart, one foot slightly behind the other. Be sure you feel very steady and balanced. Hold the barbell down against your thighs with an overhand grip, palms facing your legs. Your hands should be exactly shoulder width apart (see start).

With your arms straight or just slightly bent at the elbows, lift the bar out in front of you until it is at shoulder height (see midpoint). Keep your back straight and don't let your body sway back and forth. Concentrate on allowing only your shoulders to do the work.

Slowly lower the bar back to your thighs. Do not lower it too quickly; you want to work your shoulders on the way down, too. Repeat the motion until your set is complete.

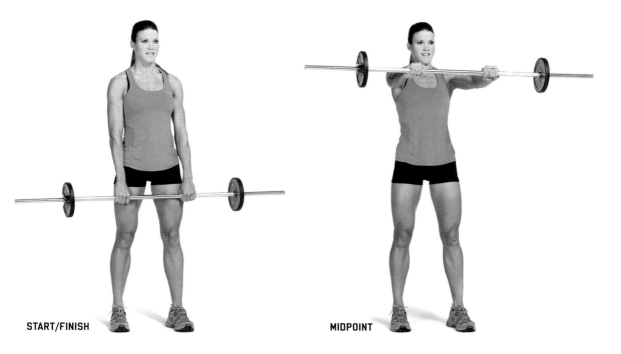

START/FINISH   **MIDPOINT**

Bench Press

The bench press may seem like an unlikely exercise for cycling, but if you were to flip it over, you would be pressing down instead of up. When riding, you are essentially pushing down on the handlebars all the time, so the bench press trains all the muscles involved in the upper body while cycling.

Lie down on the bench on your back and keep your feet flat on the floor. (You may have seen people put their feet on the bench, but that creates an unstable and dangerous position.) Place your hands on the bar approximately shoulder width apart. Positioning the hands wider than shoulder width decreases the effectiveness of this exercise, and a narrower grip will make the triceps work too much. Although there will probably be small marking rings around the bar, ignore them; they are for reference only. Be sure your hands are an equal distance from the middle of the bar.

Lift the bar off its resting hooks and hover it over your chest. Don't let it move over your head or down over your stomach. There is a point at which your arms will be perfectly vertical and the bar will feel relatively light (see start). Inhale deeply, and slowly lower the bar toward your chest while allowing your elbows to move out away from your body (see midpoint). Keep the bar away from your head and neck! The bar shouldn't touch your chest—within an inch or so is perfect.

While exhaling, push the bar back up until your arms are straight again. As you push, move the bar in a straight line. If you feel the bar moving more toward your head or stomach, make adjustments to keep it positioned over your chest. Finish your reps until the set is complete.

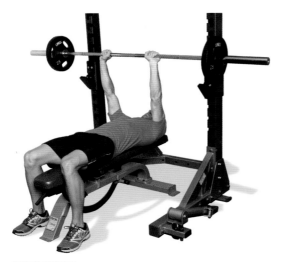

START/FINISH

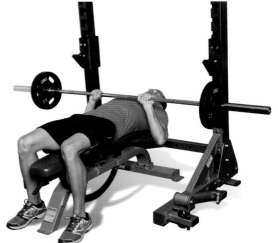

MIDPOINT

Overhand Curl

MUSCLE FOCUS biceps, wrist extensors

This exercise again targets the forearms, strengthening them for both holding your arms straight and keeping your wrists strong.

Stand with your feet apart, with one foot slightly in front of the other. Hold a barbell with an overhand grip, palms facing down or toward your legs. Your grip should be evenly spaced on the barbell, slightly wider than shoulder width. Rest the barbell against the front of your thighs, arms relaxed (see start).

Keep a very tight grip on the barbell, and keep your elbows next to your sides. Curl the barbell up to your shoulders, just under your chin (see midpoint). Slowly lower it back to rest on your thighs. Repeat the movement to complete the set.

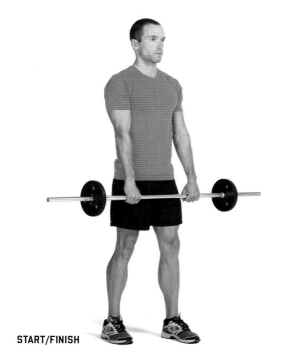

START/FINISH

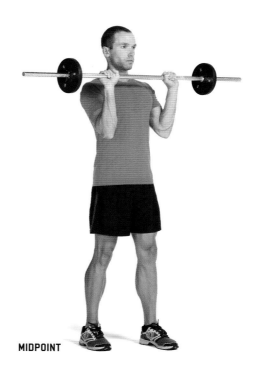

MIDPOINT

CHAPTER 12

Lower-Body Exercises for Cycling

It doesn't matter how lightweight and aerodynamic your bike is if your body doesn't have the muscle to propel it forward. Pedaling is a very unusual motor pattern because opposite sides of the body are using opposing muscle groups simultaneously. While one leg is pushing down on the pedal, the other is pulling up. So your glutes, quadriceps, and calf muscles are working on one side, while the hamstrings, hip flexors, and dorsiflexors (front of the lower leg) are working on the other side. This unique motor pattern requires equally unique exercises. Most lower-body exercises work both legs at the same time, using the same muscles on each leg, so they aren't cycling-specific enough for your needs. Most of the exercises in this chapter were designed to mimic part of the cycling movement one leg at a time. It will take longer to finish each of these exercises because you will have to do twice as many sets in order to work both legs, so account for the extra time when planning your workouts.

Walking Lunge

MUSCLE FOCUS calves, glutes, quads

The lunge allows you to focus on the pushing part of your cycling stroke. This exercise puts the leg in almost the same position as when you are on the bike and requires you to achieve full extension to get back to the start position. In addition, it alternates left and right legs, just as cycling does.

Find an open space where you have a clear path in front of you. Start by standing with your feet slightly apart, holding a dumbbell in each hand, arms at your sides (see start). Take a large step forward with one foot. As your foot lands, bend both knees to absorb the impact. Your back knee should move toward the floor but not quite touch it (see midpoint). (Touching your knee to the floor puts most of your body weight on the knee-cap, which is not a good idea.) The dumbbells should remain at your sides. Push up with both legs, bringing your back foot forward to meet your front foot.

Now step forward with your other foot, and continue taking lunging steps until you have completed your set.

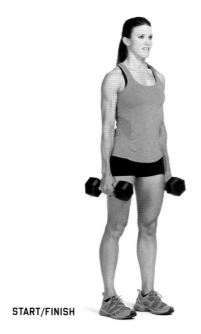

START/FINISH

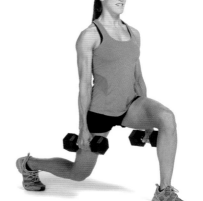

MIDPOINT (L)

One-Leg Squat

The one-leg squat is a very difficult exercise that provides amazing results once you get the hang of it. The depth of the squat is more than you will see on your bike, but it allows the muscles to get stronger and better able to handle the bike range of motion.

Stand next to an exercise machine, doorway, or something you can hold on to with one hand. Standing on the outside leg, lift the inside leg out in front and hold it (see start). Slowly bend your hip and knee, lowering yourself toward the floor. As you descend, continue to hold the other leg off the floor, and move your free arm out to your side for balance (see midpoint). Go down as far as you can or until your supporting thigh is parallel to the floor. Now push back up with the supporting leg until you are standing again. Repeat until your set is complete, then face the other direction, switch legs, and do another set. Complete 2 sets of 10 reps on each side.

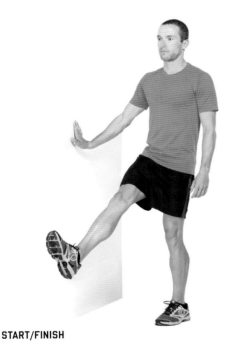

START/FINISH

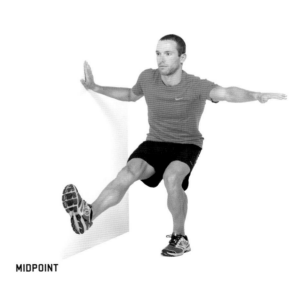

MIDPOINT

Step-up

MUSCLE FOCUS calves, glutes, quads

The step-up also focuses on the push portion of the pedal stroke, but now you have to lift your entire body weight up against the force of gravity. In addition, because you are standing upright and not bent over as you would be on the bike, the quads have to work more, making them even stronger. For this exercise, you can use any height of step you want, but something about knee-height is ideal. You can check the proper height by putting one foot on top of the step and checking to see if the upper leg is nearly parallel to the floor. A step that puts your knee higher than your hip when your foot is on it is too tall and could cause a knee injury; a shorter step is safer.

Stand about 6 to 12 inches back from the step. (Standing too far away will cause you to use forward momentum to get up on the step.) Holding a dumbbell in each hand with your arms at your sides, place one foot on top

of the step, making sure your entire foot is on the step so your heel is not hanging off the edge (see start).

To begin the step-up, transfer all your body weight onto the foot on top of the step and use the muscles in that leg to push yourself up (see midpoint). It will be temping to use the other leg, specifically your calf muscles, to push off the ground, but that diminishes the effectiveness of this exercise. Your goal is to have the foot leave the ground flat-footed; that is, your heel and toes will leave the ground at the same time. Once both feet are on top of the step, step down with the working leg, keeping the other leg on the step.

Now complete the rep by again pushing up with the leg that is on the step. Step down and continue alternating, pushing up and stepping down with each leg, until your set is complete.

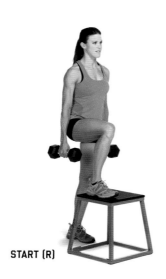

START (R)

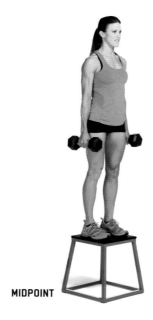

MIDPOINT

Lying Hip Flex

MUSCLE FOCUS dorsiflexors, hamstrings, hip flexors

This is one of only a few exercises that train the recovery portion of the bike stroke. The low-pulley machine mimics the effect of having your foot clipped into the bike pedal and lets you work the muscles that pull the pedal back to the top of the stroke.

Lie on your back in front of a low-pulley machine, with your feet toward the machine. Prop yourself up on your elbows if that's more comfortable. Hook the ankle strap over the toes of one foot far enough so that it won't slip off (see start). Make sure there isn't any slack in the cable in this position.

Pull back with your toes to make the weight stack rise a little. Keeping your toes pointed up and flexed back, pull your knee toward your chest (see midpoint). The other leg should remain on the floor. Slowly return your leg to the start position and repeat until your set is done, then switch legs to do another set.

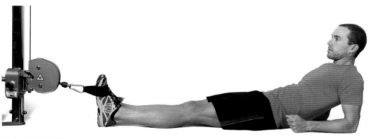

START/FINISH

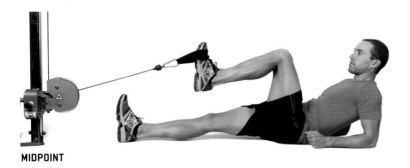

MIDPOINT

Knee Raise

Knee raises also work the muscle required for pulling your foot back to the top of the stroke, but instead of using a machine, this exercise requires that you lift your own body weight. As a sidenote, knee raises have often been considered an abdominal exercise, which they are not. Simply put, in order for the abdominals to work, the spine has to flex, because that's what the abdominals are designed to do. There is no spinal flexion during a knee raise, so there is no abdominal action.

There are specific exercise benches made for this exercise, or you can use the arms of a dip machine or straps that allow you to hang from your arms. Position yourself on the equipment so that you are supported by your arms and your legs hang freely (see start).

Pull both knees up toward your chest as high as you can (see midpoint). Slowly allow them to return toward the ground, and as soon as your legs are straight, lift them again. As a variation, you can alternate lifting one leg at a time, in a cycling-type movement (one leg is coming up while the other is going down). You can add ankle weights to make this exercise more difficult. Complete 3 sets of 25 reps.

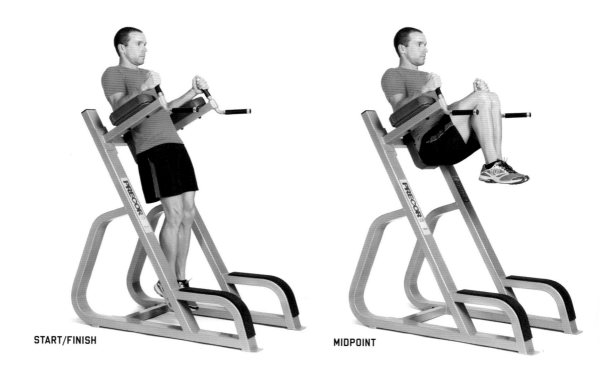

START/FINISH　　　　　　　　**MIDPOINT**

Single-Calf Raise

The single-calf raise is more specific for cycling because while one leg is pushing, the other is pulling, so only one side of your body is using your calf muscles at a time. You can do this exercise standing on the floor, but it is more effective to stand on the edge of a step, curb, aerobics bench, or even a board.

Stand with the balls of your feet on the edge of the step so your heels are hanging off the back. Place the foot of your resting leg behind the ankle of the working leg. Drop the heel of your working leg down as far as you can to maximize the exercise (see start). Hold on to something to help with balance.

Push up on the ball of your foot as high as you can (see midpoint). Slowly return to the start position and repeat 15 to 25 reps to complete a set. Complete another set with the other leg and continue alternating legs until you have done 3 sets on each side.

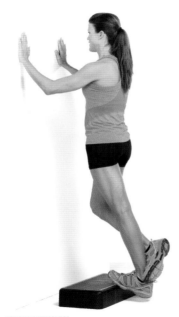

START/FINISH

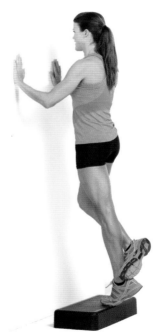

MIDPOINT

Single-Leg Extension

MUSCLE FOCUS quads

The single-leg extension is cycling specific because only one leg is extending at a time. Just as with the regular leg extension exercise, if you have knee problems, it is better to skip this exercise; but if your knees are healthy, you should be fine.

Sit down on a leg extension machine and line up your knees with the machine's pivot point. On some machines, this requires adjusting the seat back. The pivot point is evident (or can be found on the machine's instruction card) and is usually at the edge of the seat. If your knees are too far forward, there will be a lot of strain on them at the start of the exercise. Place your feet behind the footpad and adjust it so the pad rests just above your feet, on your shins (see start). (Some machines

adjust themselves, so you may not have to do this.) If you can adjust how far under the seat the leg pad is, move it so that you start with your knees bent at about a 90-degree angle. A sharper angle at the start can cause knee pain, especially if you have had a prior knee injury.

Hold on to the handles and straighten out one leg as far as possible (see midpoint). Keep the other leg in place, hanging down in a relaxed position. Slowly lower your leg back down to a point just before the weight stack comes to a rest, then repeat until your set is complete. Now do a set with the other leg. Continue alternating legs until all your sets are done.

CAUTION: If your knees hurt at all during this exercise, skip it and use another exercise for the quadriceps.

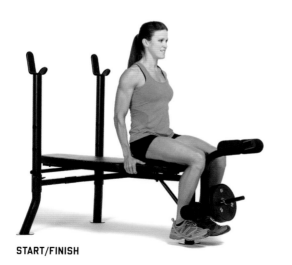

START/FINISH

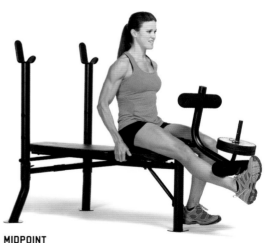

MIDPOINT

Seated Leg Curl

The seated leg curl is more specific to cycling than the lying leg curl because it places your hips in the flexed position similar to your position on the bike. This allows your hamstrings to start in a slightly stretched position, as occurs while cycling.

Sit on the seated leg curl machine and adjust the seat back so your knees line up with the machine's pivot point. The seat is usually quite short on these machines and may stop about halfway to your knees, so be sure to identify the proper pivot point. Put your feet and legs on top of the leg pad. Adjust the leg pad so it is in contact with your Achilles tendon and not pushing

on your feet. (Some machines automatically adjust the foot pad, so you may not have to do this.) If there is a thigh pad, lower it until it makes contact and is snug against your thighs. If your knees rise during the exercise, you will have to adjust this pad downward (see start).

Hold on to the hand grips and bend your knees, pulling your feet down and under the seat as far as you can. At the end of the pull, give an extra squeeze to go a little farther (see midpoint). Slowly straighten your legs back out until the weight stack almost touches down, then start another rep. Continue reps until your set is complete.

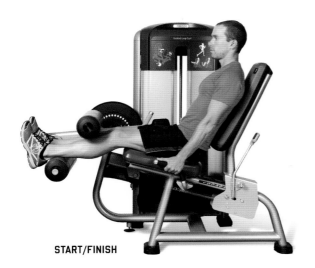

START/FINISH

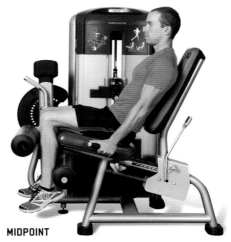

MIDPOINT

Toe Taps

Toe taps are an unusual exercise that you won't see many people doing because it doesn't look like an exercise, and there is no weight involved. When you are pulling the pedal back to the top of a stroke, your ankle has to flex in order to pull your toes up. While this is a small movement, it is very important. The dorsiflexor muscles keep your toes from dropping, and when they get tired, you can't pull very effectively on the pedals.

Sit on a chair or bench that is at a height that allows your thighs to be parallel with the floor; when the height is not correct, the exercise is less effective. Place your feet flat on the floor, positioning your heels directly under your knees and your feet together (see start).

Now tap your toes, alternating left and right foot, lifting your toes as high as you can while keeping your heels on the floor, and as fast as you can for as long as you can—up to 60 seconds (see midpoint). This is a muscular endurance exercise so we aren't counting reps, just time. After a set, rest for 1 minute and repeat two more times.

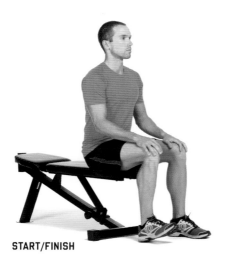

START/FINISH

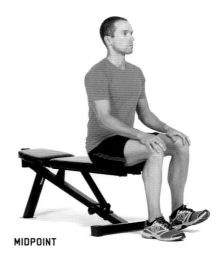

MIDPOINT

Dumbbell Deep Squat

MUSCLE FOCUS glutes, hamstrings, quads

The dumbbell deep squat uses both legs simultaneously, but you will focus on contracting the muscles in only one leg at a time. This takes both balance and strength, and it allows you to move through a large range of motion.

Stand with your feet about 4 to 5 inches apart, with your toes turned out slightly. Hold a dumbbell in each hand, with your arms straight and your palms facing your thighs (see start). Keep your arms relaxed at your sides during the entire movement.

Slowly bend down as if you were going to set the dumbbells on the ground beside your feet. As you squat, bend both your knees and hips at the same time. Your hips should move out behind you, and your shoulders should

lean forward. Really concentrate on keeping your back as straight as possible, your head up and eyes forward. Squat until your hips are slightly lower than your knees (see midpoint). The dumbbells may or may not touch the floor, depending on how long your arms are. Now shift your weight to one leg and concentrate on pushing back up to the standing position using the muscles in just one leg. Don't lift the other foot off the ground; it's there to help you balance and provide a little push if you need it. As you stand back up, raise your hips and shoulders at the same time, keeping your head up and eyes forward. Repeat this movement until you complete the set, then do a set with the opposite leg.

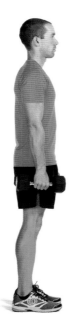

START/FINISH

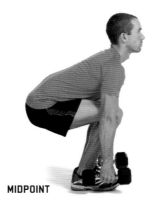

MIDPOINT

Reverse Lunge

MUSCLE FOCUS glutes, hamstrings, quads

The reverse lunge is very similar to the forward lunge except that the leg doing the most work is the one behind you instead of the one in front of you. The leg stepping back experiences a lot of eccentric contraction, while the front leg concentrically contracts—similar to what happens when you ride.

Stand with your feet a few inches apart, holding a dumbbell in each hand down at your sides, palms facing your legs (see start). Allow the dumbbells to hang down throughout the exercise; they simply add weight to the lunge, not arm movement.

Take a big step back with one foot as if you were stepping backward over a puddle. Land with only your toes touching the floor, then bend both knees until the back knee is about an inch from the floor (see midpoint). As you are bending down, keep your upper body erect; do not bend at the waist. Once you are at the bottom of the movement, push with both legs simultaneously and with enough force to propel yourself back to the start position. You have to push hard enough so that your back foot does not drag on the floor, but not so hard as to force a step forward. Repeat with the opposite leg, alternating left and right steps until your set is complete.

CAUTION: This exercise can be hard on the knees if you don't take a big enough step. Monitor your front knee—if it travels forward past your toes, you didn't take a big enough step back, so your body is having to move forward to complete the lunge.

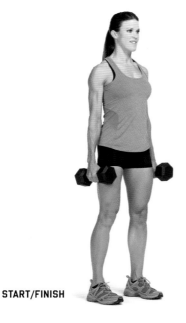

START/FINISH

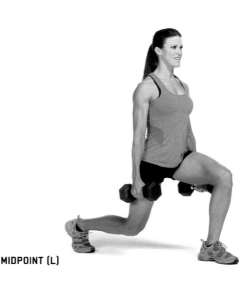

MIDPOINT (L)

CHAPTER 13

Upper-Body Exercises for Running

There is an old saying among track coaches that you can only run as fast as you can move your arms. This sounds odd, but the arms and legs do move together while you are running. The pumping of your arms acts as a counterbalance to your legs to help rotate your hips and torso. Ever try running with your arms down at your sides? You can't move very fast, and it feels awkward.

Keeping your arms pumping takes muscle. The elbows are bent, which requires the biceps muscles to work, and the entire arm moves forward and back, requiring the shoulders, chest, and back muscles to work. And the up-and-down motion of running causes your shoulders to bounce, which must be stabilized by the surrounding muscles to prevent injury. Over long distances your upper body can become tired, so the more strength and muscular endurance it has, the better.

The upper-body muscles covered in this chapter include the biceps, which keep the elbows bent; the triceps, which extend the elbows and balance the biceps; the deltoids, which move the arms fore and aft; and the lats, trapezius, and rhomboids, which stabilize the shoulder movements.

Hammer Curl

The hammer curl is specific for running because it places the hand in a neutral position, just as it is while you are running and holding your elbows bent. The neutral hand position changes the emphasis of the exercise from the biceps brachii muscle to the brachioradialis muscle (both help bend the elbow), which is used more when you hold your arms in a bent position while running.

Stand with your feet shoulder width apart, one foot slightly in front of the other. Hold a dumbbell in each hand, arms straight and relaxed at your sides, palms facing your thighs (see start).

Keeping one arm at rest, with the other arm pull the dumbbell up to your shoulder by bending your elbow (see midpoint). Keep your elbow at your side when you lift the dumbbell; only your forearm and hand should be moving. Slowly let the dumbbell back down to the start position, completely straightening the arm, then repeat with the other arm. Alternate left and right curls until your set is complete.

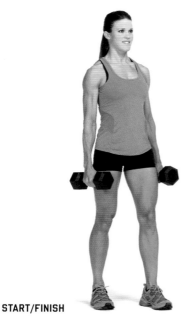

START/FINISH

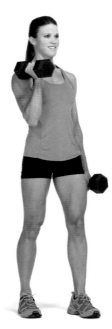

MIDPOINT (R)

Runner's Raise

The runner's raise trains the biceps and the front part of the shoulder to keep your hands up by your sides during a long run. When you lack strength in these areas, you will notice that your arms slowly drop down as you run, reducing your efficiency.

Stand with your feet apart, one foot slightly in front of the other. Hold a dumbbell in each hand. Keeping your elbows at your sides, bend your arms to bring the dumbbells up in front of you until your arms are at a

90-degree angle (see start). (This is basically the halfway point of a hammer curl.)

Holding the 90-degree angle of your arms, lift your elbows forward and up until they are pointing straight out in front of you (see midpoint). The dumbbells will finish the movement near your head. Slowly lower your arms until your elbows come back to your sides (the dumbbells are still being held up in front of you), and repeat until your set is complete.

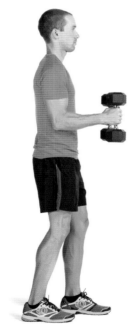

START/FINISH

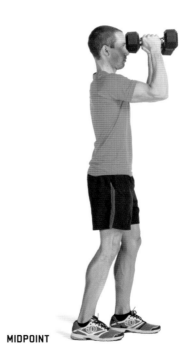

MIDPOINT

Upright Row

MUSCLE FOCUS biceps, delts, trapezius

The upright row assists in making the shoulders stronger (mainly the top of the shoulder), and with the trapezius prevents your shoulders from bouncing during your run, which can cause fatigue and injury.

Hold a dumbbell in each hand with your arms straight down in front of you and your palms facing your legs (see start). Stand with your feet shoulder width apart.

Pull the dumbbells up in a straight line, following the front of your torso until they reach your chin (see midpoint). Your elbows should end up pointed out to your sides or slightly upward. The key is to keep the dumbbells really close to your body and your elbows above your wrists at all times. If you pretend there are strings attached to your elbows that are being pulled from above, the motion will be very smooth. Slowly lower the dumbbells back down to the starting position and repeat until your set is complete.

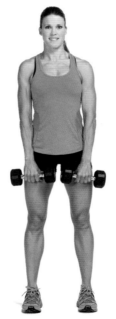

START/FINISH

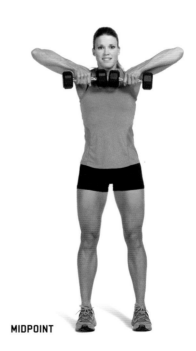

MIDPOINT

Shrug

The shrug helps keep your shoulders high and able to hold the weight of your arms without bouncing.

Stand with your feet together. Hold a dumbbell in each hand with your palms facing your thighs and your arms hanging down straight at your sides. Let your shoulders sag, allowing the weight of the dumbbells to pull them down (see start).

Keeping your arms straight, lift your shoulders up toward your ears, effectively shrugging your shoulders (see midpoint). Do not move your shoulders forward or backward or rotate them in a circle—the movement is straight up and down. Slowly lower your shoulders back into the sagging start position and repeat the movement until your set is done.

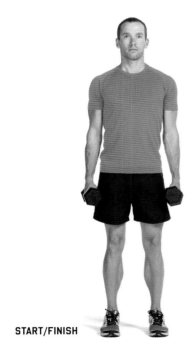

START/FINISH

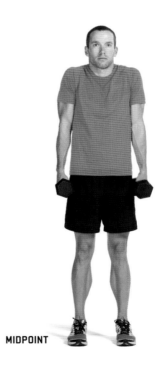

MIDPOINT

Retraction

If you have ever felt your upper back become fatigued during a run or found yourself needing to stretch your shoulders while running, this exercise will help. By working the back of the shoulder, retraction helps keep your torso upright and prevents slouching.

Attach your resistance tubing to the door anchor or wrap it around a pole a couple of feet off the floor. Sit down on the floor facing the anchor. Hold one handle in each hand with your arms straight out in front of you. Scoot back until the tubing is pulling you forward. Let your shoulders relax so that the tubing is pulling your shoulders forward and your back is rounded (see start).

Keeping your body still and your arms straight, pull your shoulders back while pushing your chest out (see midpoint). Attempt to squeeze your shoulder blades together, feeling the increased resistance on the tubing. This is a small movement but an important one for the trapezius muscle.

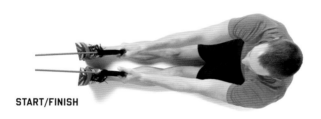

START/FINISH

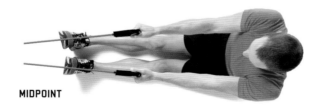

MIDPOINT

Tubing Row

MUSCLE FOCUS biceps, delts, lats

If you have ever seen someone running with flailing arms, then you'll understand why this exercise is important. The tubing row teaches you to pull your arms up tight against your body, improving efficiency and aerodynamics while also strengthening your shoulders (mainly the back of the shoulder) and back.

Attach your resistance tubing to the door anchor or wrap it around a pole at shoulder height. Hold one handle in each hand. Facing the anchor, hold your arms straight out in front of you, palms facing together and step back until the tubing is pulling you forward (see start). Stand with your feet apart and one foot slightly in front of the other to prevent you from being pulled forward. Keep your body upright and your back straight.

Pull back on the tubing with both hands, trying to bring your hands all the way to the sides of your body (see midpoint). In this position, your arms and hands should be in approximately the same position as they are when you run. Slowly let your arms back out until they are straight again. If there isn't enough resistance, step back a little farther to make the tubing tighter. Repeat until your set is complete.

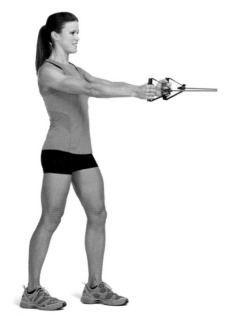

START/FINISH

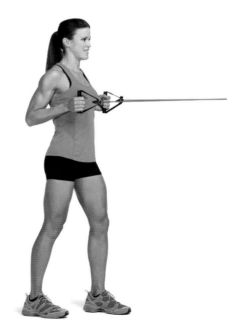

MIDPOINT

Barbell Lift

The barbell lift trains your biceps and delts while necessitating an upright stance, such as you would have during a run. This exercise can't be done hunched over, so it engages the delts to pull and maintain shoulder stability while the biceps are working—just as happens during a run.

Stand with your feet shoulder width apart. Hold a barbell against your thighs with an overhand grip, palms facing toward your legs. Your grip should be slightly narrower than shoulder width, with hands evenly spaced from the center (see start).

Keeping your elbows out to the sides, pull the bar up in front of your body until it's directly under your chin (see midpoint). Throughout the lift, the bar should stay close to your body, while your elbows should be higher than your wrists, and your wrists should be higher than the bar. Slowly lower the bar back down the front of your body until your arms are completely straight again. Repeat until your set is complete.

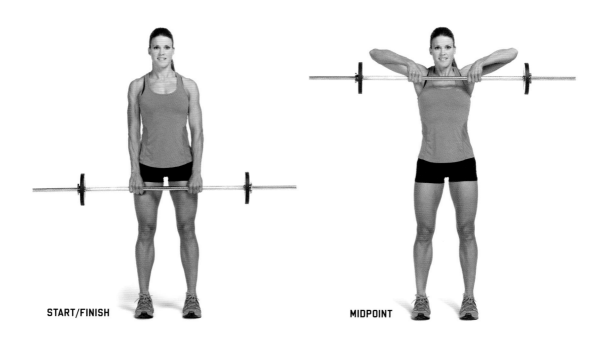

START/FINISH   MIDPOINT

Barbell Row

MUSCLE FOCUS biceps, delts, erector spinae, lats

The barbell row works the biceps, delts, and lats to move the barbell, but it also engages the erector spinae in the lower back to keep you stable in a bent-over position. This strengthens the lower back, which is what keeps you upright and not hunched over during a run.

Hold on to a barbell with a shoulder-width, overhand grip (palms facing your body). Bend your knees slightly, and bend forward at the waist about 45 to 60 degrees while keeping your back straight (see start). Relax your arms and let the weight hang straight down.

While holding this position and keeping your back straight, use just your arms to pull the bar up toward the bottom of your ribs (see midpoint). Try to get the bar to touch your lower chest. Slowly lower the bar back down until your arms are straight. Pay close attention to your lower back during this exercise and keep it as straight as possible—slouching or rounding it can cause injury. Also take care to pull the weight up slowly; do not jerk it up. The rest of your body should be stationary as you repeat the movement to finish your set.

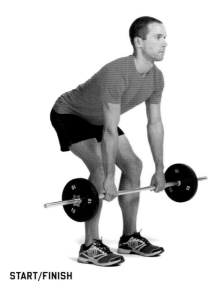

START/FINISH

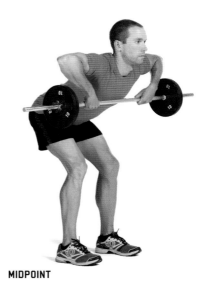

MIDPOINT

Dumbbell French Curl

It may not seem like the triceps are working while running because you don't actively push down on anything; but when you train the biceps, the triceps are stabilizing the elbow joint. Strengthening them helps you maintain a balance in the arm.

Lie on your back on an exercise bench with your feet flat on the floor. Hold a dumbbell in one hand up over your chest and shoulder, parallel to your body, with your arm fully extended. Place your other hand on your arm just below your elbow, using it to steady and support your lifting arm (see start).

Bend your elbow and slowly lower the dumbbell until it is beside your head, about ear level (see midpoint). Your supporting hand should keep your elbow from moving. Use your triceps to straighten your arm, raising the dumbbell back to the starting position. Repeat until your reps are complete. Switch arms and do the same number of reps on the opposite side to complete your set.

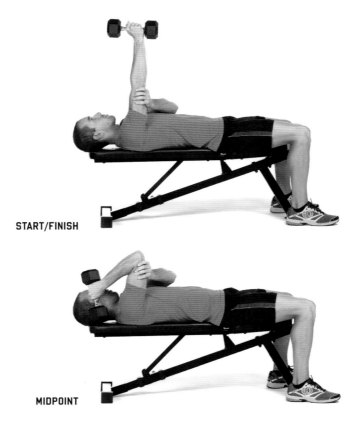

START/FINISH

MIDPOINT

CHAPTER 14

Lower-Body Exercises for Running

By the time you get to the run portion of a triathlon, your legs have done a lot of work and are probably starting to fatigue. Fortunately, strength training can give you the extra muscular strength and endurance you need to keep moving in the late stages of a race.

During the run, your legs are working in opposing directions. While one leg is moving back to provide propulsion, the other leg is recovering from the stride and moving forward to start the next stride. This is all done through a very complex motor pattern enlisting the coordination of several muscles. The glutes, quadriceps, hamstrings, and calves are all large muscle groups, so it is important to work each of them in turn, as well as all together. Although there is disagreement about which lower-body muscle group is most important during a run, here we assume they are all equally important and should be worked accordingly.

The running stride is divided into two parts, the push and the recovery, which use different lower-body muscles. The push is what propels you forward, and it begins when your foot hits the ground in front of you and ends when you lift your foot off the ground to start the recovery. The recovery begins when your foot leaves the ground, continues as your foot travels back in front of you, and ends when your heel hits the ground to start the next push. The muscles involved in the push include the glutes for hip extension, the hamstrings for hip extension and knee flexion, and the calves for plantar flexion (pushing off). The muscles involved in the recovery include the hip flexors to bring the thigh forward again, the quadriceps for knee extension, and the shin muscles for dorsiflexion (lifting the toes so you can land heel first).

Split Squat

MUSCLE FOCUS calves, glutes, hamstrings, quads

The split squat is unusual in that while both legs are bending and extending, they are doing so in different ranges of motion, and while the same muscles are being used in each leg, they are engaged at different intensities. This is similar to what happens when you change your stride length when running—the same muscles are working, but in different ranges and intensities. The range of motion for each leg is greater than you will encounter in your running stride, but it teaches your legs to be able to handle an increased stress.

Holding a dumbbell in each hand with your palms facing your thighs, stand with your feet together. Take a big step forward with one leg (see start).

Bend both knees simultaneously so that your back knee moves toward the floor and your front knee moves toward your toes. Your front knee may move past your toes during this exercise: The deeper bend at the knee will provide greater results, and because the effort is split between front and back legs, there is little danger of placing too much stress on the knee. However, if you have had a posterior cruciate ligament injury, you should step out farther to keep your knee behind your toes. Keep your torso upright and straight; do not lean forward. Stop when your back knee is about an inch from the floor (see midpoint). Push against the floor with both feet to rise back up to the start position. The dumbbells should remain hanging at your sides the entire time, which allows your legs to do all of the work. Repeat until your reps are done, take a 30-second rest, then step forward with the other leg and do the same number of reps to complete the set.

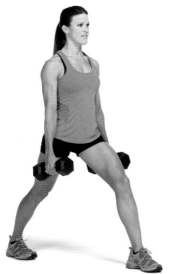

START/FINISH

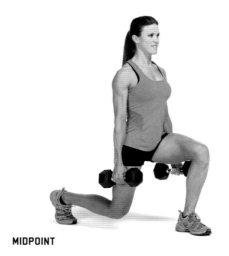

MIDPOINT

Squat

MUSCLE FOCUS calves, glutes, hamstrings, quads

Although you do not bend your hips and knees as far while running as you do during the squat, the increased range of motion of this exercise gives the leg muscles a large buffer of strength for the push that propels you forward. The squat is one of the greatest exercises for the lower body, but also one of the most dangerous. It should be performed inside a squat cage for maximum safety. The squat cage has two upright bars that hold the barbell in place while you load the bar with weight and a pair of safety catch bars that are there in case you can't get back up from the low position. Adjust the catch bars so they are just below the level the barbell will reach at the lowest point of the squat.

With the barbell resting on the cage, duck under it and position yourself so it rests across the top of your shoulders, just below your neck. If this is uncomfortable, wrap the bar with a towel for extra padding. Stand up with the barbell, take a small step back, and position your feet shoulder width apart, toes slightly turned out (see start).

Inhale deeply and hold your breath as you descend. Holding your breath creates intra-abdominal pressure, which helps to support your lumbar spine during the descent. Keeping your back straight, bend your knees and hips simultaneously to begin the descent. As you squat, move your hips out behind you and your shoulders forward (see alternate view). Be sure to keep the barbell directly over your feet during the entire movement. Squat until your thighs are parallel to the floor (see midpoint)—any less is a partial squat and is less effective. Exhale as you push your feet into the floor and stand back up. As you stand, be sure to lift your hips and shoulders at the same time, not one then the other. Repeat the movement until your set is complete.

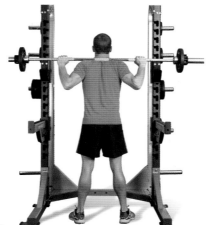

START/FINISH

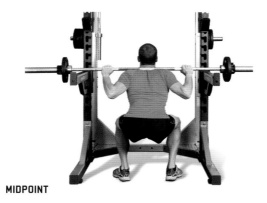

MIDPOINT

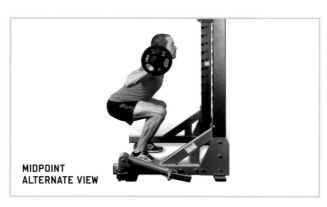

MIDPOINT
ALTERNATE VIEW

Cable Hip Flex

You don't run just by pushing off the ground; your leg has to recover and move into position for the next step. Because your leg moves through the air there is little resistance, but the muscles still have to lift the weight of your leg. The cable hip flex exercise works the hip flexors and quadriceps muscles responsible for the recovery phase.

Attach the ankle strap of a low-pulley cable machine to one leg. (As an alternative, you can also put your toes through a single-handle strap.) Face away from the machine and stand

far enough out to create resistance on the cable. Hold on to something for balance if necessary. The working leg should begin slightly behind you (see start).

Keeping your leg straight and your toes pointed up, slowly raise your leg out in front of you, as high as you can (see midpoint). Don't try to kick or use momentum to get your leg up higher. Slowly lower your leg back to the start position and repeat until your reps are finished, then switch legs and do the same number of reps on the other side to complete your set.

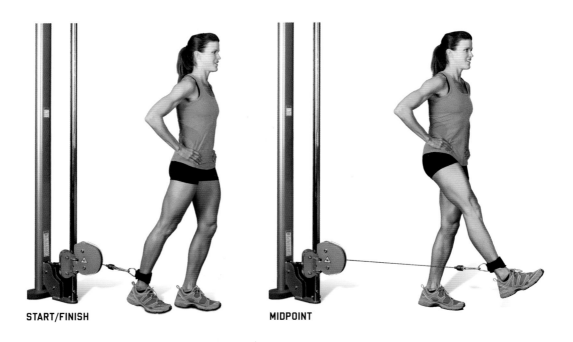

START/FINISH   MIDPOINT

Standing Leg Curl

The standing leg curl is the most specific hamstring exercise for running because it places you in the same position you are in while running: standing up.

Attach an ankle weight to each leg. If you need more resistance, wrap a second ankle weight over the first. Stand facing something you can hold on to for balance (see start).

Lift the toes of one foot off the floor, then bend your knee to bring that foot up behind you (see midpoint). Keep your upper leg parallel to the wall. Pretend you are trying to kick yourself in the buttocks, but not hard or fast. As you lift the foot, do not lean forward; keep your torso upright and straight. Lift the foot as high as you can in a controlled manner. Lower the foot back to the floor and repeat until your reps are done. Switch to the other leg and do the same number of reps to complete the set. Do 3 sets of 15 reps with each leg.

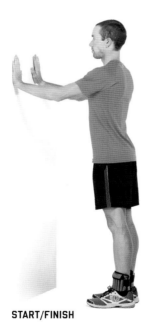

START/FINISH

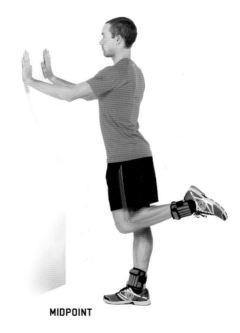

MIDPOINT

Lying Single-Leg Curl

The lying single-leg curl makes each leg work independently and allows you to use more weight so you can get more individualized results and improve your running.

Find the pivot point of the lying leg-curl machine, usually at the edge of the padding. Stand at the end of the bench with your knees right against the padding and lie on your stomach, holding on to the handles (see start). (Some machines have pads for your elbows to rest on; others have a flat bench to rest your chest and head on.) Your kneecaps should hang off the end of the bench and be lined up with the machine pivot point, and your feet should be underneath the leg pad. Some machines adjust this automatically, but if not, adjust it so it is in contact with the back of your lower legs (on your Achilles tendon) and is not pushing on your foot.

Keeping one leg relaxed and in the start position, pull the leg pad as far up as you can with the other leg (see midpoint). The goal is to get the pad all the way to your buttocks. The farther you can curl your leg, the more you will get out of this exercise. Slowly lower the leg, then repeat until your reps are complete. Switch legs and do the same number of reps to complete the set.

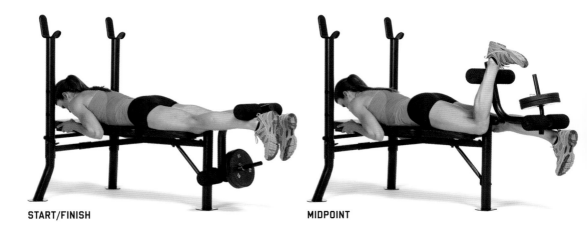

START/FINISH   MIDPOINT

Cable Toe Raise

The cable toe raise focuses on the dorsiflexor muscles in your shin, which are responsible for lifting your toes during the recovery. If these muscles are weak, you will shuffle your feet instead of efficiently pushing off the ground with each foot strike.

Sit on the floor facing a low-pulley machine. Place the toes of one foot through a single-handle strap attached to the cable. Scoot yourself back until the cable is pulling your toes toward the machine (see start). You can lean back, resting on your elbows or your hands.

Pull your toes toward you as far as you can, then slowly release them back toward the machine (see midpoint). This is a small movement of the foot that you will feel rather acutely in your shin muscles. Complete all your reps on that foot, then switch and do the same number of reps on the other foot to complete the set.

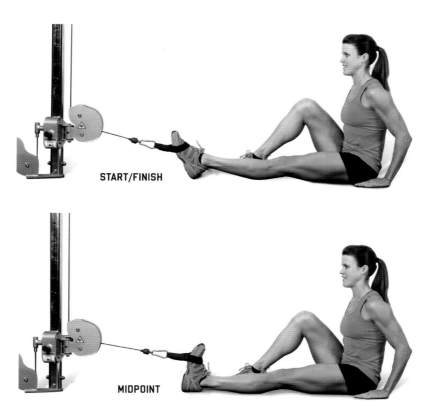

START/FINISH

MIDPOINT

Seated Toe Raise

The seated toe raise focuses on the shin muscles, but both feet are working together, and with the knees bent, the body has to work harder to move a light weight.

Place a weight plate (25 to 45 pounds) on the floor in front of a chair or bench. Sitting on the edge of the chair or bench, move the plate so that your heels are on the edge of the plate and your toes hang off the end. Put your feet together and keep your heels directly under your knees so your toes are in front of your knees. Place another weight plate on your toes and hold it there with both hands. If this is uncomfortable on your toes, place a folded towel between your toes and the plate as extra padding. Allow your toes to drop to the floor and relax (see start).

Lift the toes of both feet as high as you can, lifting the weight plate toward the ceiling (see midpoint). You can rock back on your heels, but don't move your upper body or legs; only your feet and ankles should move. Lower your toes back to the floor and repeat until the set is complete.

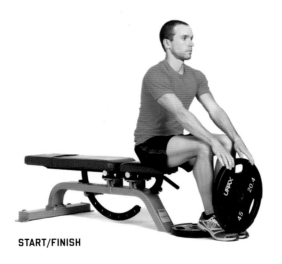

START/FINISH

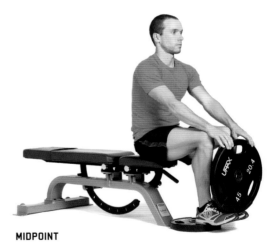

MIDPOINT

Leg Press

MUSCLE FOCUS calves, glutes, hamstrings, quads

The leg press is really just a squat in a seated position and offers the same benefits as the squat, but it is safer because there is no weight on your shoulders; instead, it moves through your hips.

Position your feet on the platform of the leg press machine, spaced slightly wider than shoulder width, with your toes pointed out slightly. Be sure to keep your feet completely on the platform; don't let your heels hang off the bottom. Adjust the seat until your knees are bent at about 90 degrees. An angle greater than 90 degrees will put too much strain on the knees, whereas an angle of less than 90 degrees will decrease the effective-ness of the exercise. If the machine allows you to adjust the back rest, make it comfortable. Place your hands on the handles down at your sides (see start).

Push against the platform with both feet at the same time. When you push, put equal pressure on your heels and the balls of your feet. Don't allow the focus to be on your toes—that would make this a calf exercise. Push until your legs are not quite straight (see midpoint). Do not lock your knees! Slowly bend your legs, letting the platform move back toward you. When the weight stack is close to touching down, repeat the movement until your set is finished.

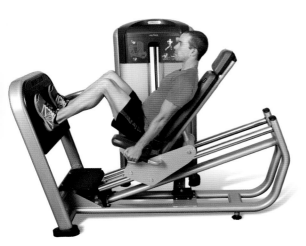

START/FINISH

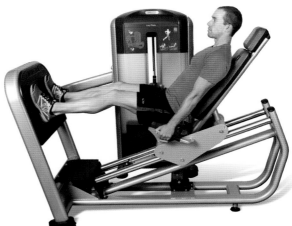

MIDPOINT

Romanian Deadlift

The Romanian deadlift is actually not a dead-lift at all since you're neither picking up the weight from the floor nor putting it back down to the floor with each rep. In fact, when done correctly, this exercise doesn't involve the quads in the way a deadlift does, but instead focuses on hip extension via the hamstrings and glutes—exactly what you need for a powerful running stride.

This exercise requires a barbell be loaded with weight and set at a starting height that is about waist high. If you're using a heavy weight, use a power rack or squat rack to set up. Hold the bar slightly wider than shoulder width using an overhand grip (palms facing the legs). Pick the bar up and step away from the rack. Your feet should still be shoulder width apart and you should stand with your chest up, a slight curve in your lower back, and your knees slightly bent—not locked (see start).

Keep your lower back in the slightly curved position as you bend at the waist and allow the barbell to slide down your thighs until you feel a stretch in your hamstrings (see midpoint). If you can reach all the way down to your knees, stop there.

Once you reach your stretched position, reverse the motion and stand back up, all the while keeping your back slightly bent. All the motion should come from the waist and hips. At the top of the motion, squeeze your glutes and push your hips forward for a full contraction. Repeat the movement until your set is complete.

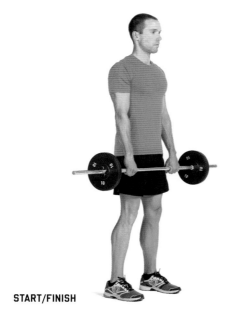

START/FINISH

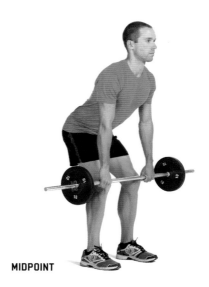

MIDPOINT

Medicine Ball Pike

This exercise works the small muscles that you use to lift your knee toward your chest, which mimics the recovery part of the running stride.

Lie on your back on the floor with a medicine ball between your feet, using one foot on each side of the ball to squeeze it and hold it in place. Prop yourself up on your elbows, and use your abdominal muscles to keep your torso straight from your hips to your shoulders—don't allow your back to sag toward the floor (see start).

Your upper body should be straight and still as you lift the ball using both legs. Keep your legs straight as you raise the ball as high as you can (see midpoint). If you can't reach this point, use a lighter medicine ball. Slowly lower the ball back down, but don't let it touch the ground. When it gets within an inch of the floor, lift it back up again, repeating your reps until the set is complete.

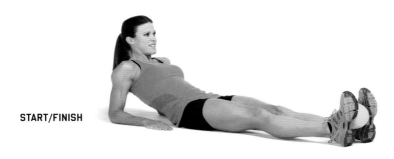

START/FINISH

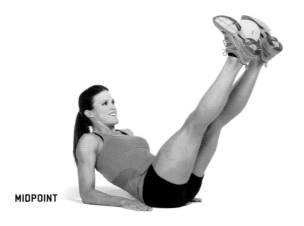

MIDPOINT

Glute Lift

This exercise involves a very small movement but requires a lot of intensity to complete it correctly—or at all—but it will pay off during the push phase of each stride, giving you more power to propel yourself forward.

Kneel facing your stability ball. To increase the intensity of this exercise, you can wear a pair of ankle weights or place a light dumbbell or medicine ball between your feet. Lie forward over the stability ball, placing your hands in front of you, shoulder width apart. Keep the stability ball right under your hips. Hold your upper body straight from the hips to the shoulders, and keep your feet together, with your legs straight out behind the stability ball, toes touching the floor (see start).

Concentrate on tightening your buttocks and lifting your legs as high as you can. Keep your legs straight and really squeeze the glutes as you lift (see midpoint). Slowly lower the legs back toward the floor, relax the glutes, and repeat to finish the set.

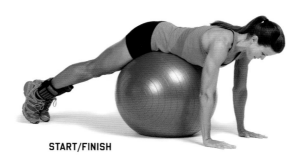

START/FINISH

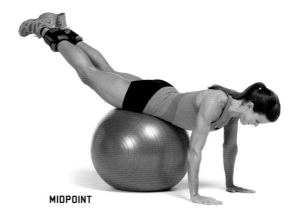

MIDPOINT

APPENDIXES

APPENDIX A

Exercise Index

Use these tables to find exercises that target specific muscle groups. Refer back to Table 6.1 (pages 68–70) to pinpoint problems that affect swimming, cycling, and running. Build your program to address your own limitations or simply build a balanced program.

The core exercises found in Chapter 8 are not included in this list because they do not target any one specific muscle group, but rather the entire torso along with muscles in the arms or legs, depending on the exercise. If you feel your core is weak, refer to Chapter 8 for more on how to integrate these exercise into your program.

	UPPER-BODY EXERCISES			
BICEPS	SWIM	BIKE	RUN	EQUIPMENT
Barbell Lift, p. 180			✔	barbell
Barbell Row, p. 181			✔	barbell
Dumbbell Curl, p. 126	✔			dumbbells
Hammer Curl, p. 174			✔	dumbbells
Overhand Curl, p. 159		✔		barbell
Runner's Raise, p. 175			✔	dumbbells
Tubing Row, p. 179			✔	tubing
Tubing Stroke, p. 123	✔			tubing
Upright Row, p. 176			✔	dumbbells

Continued

CHEST (pectorals)	SWIM	BIKE	RUN	EQUIPMENT
Bench Press, *p. 158*		✔		bench, bar, plates
Bridging Pullover, *p. 122*	✔			tubing, exercise ball
Dip, *p. 130*	✔			dip stand
Dumbbell Fly, *p. 128*	✔			dumbbells, exercise ball
Dumbbell Handle Push-up, *p. 152*		✔		dumbbells
Dumbbell Incline Press, *p. 151*		✔		dumbbells, bench
Protraction, *p. 150*		✔		tubing
Tubing Stroke, *p. 123*	✔			tubing

LOWER BACK	SWIM	BIKE	RUN	EQUIPMENT
Back Extension, *p. 149*		✔		back extension bench

SHOULDERS (deltoids, trapezius)	SWIM	BIKE	RUN	EQUIPMENT
Barbell Front Raise, *p. 157*		✔		barbell
Barbell Lift, *p. 180*			✔	barbell
Barbell Row, *p. 181*			✔	barbell
Bench Press, *p. 158*		✔		bench, bar, plates
Bridging Pullover, *p. 122*	✔			tubing, exercise ball
Dip, *p. 130*	✔			dip stand
Dumbbell Angled Raise, *p. 133*	✔			dumbbells
Dumbbell Fly, *p. 128*	✔			dumbbells, exercise ball
Dumbbell Front Raise, *p. 155*	✔			dumbbells
Dumbbell Handle Push-up, *p. 152*		✔		dumbbells
Dumbbell Incline Press, *p. 151*		✔		dumbbells, bench
Dumbbell Lateral Raise, *p. 132*	✔			dumbbells
Dumbbell Shoulder Press, *p. 124*	✔			dumbbells, exercise ball

SHOULDERS (deltoids, trapezius) Continued	SWIM	BIKE	RUN	EQUIPMENT
One-Arm Throw, *p. 120*	✔			tubing
Protraction, *p. 150*		✔		tubing
Retraction, *p. 178*			✔	tubing
Runner's Raise, *p. 175*			✔	dumbbells
Shrug, *p. 177*			✔	dumbbells
Slam Dunk, *p. 121*	✔			medicine ball
Tubing Row, *p. 179*			✔	tubing
Tubing Stroke, *p. 123*	✔			tubing
Upright Row, *p. 176*			✔	dumbbells

TRICEPS	SWIM	BIKE	RUN	EQUIPMENT
Bench Press, *p. 158*		✔		bench, bar, plates
Dip, *p. 130*	✔			dip stand
Dumbbell French Curl, *p. 182*			✔	dumbbells, bench
Dumbbell Handle Push-up, *p. 152*		✔		dumbbells
Dumbbell Incline Press, *p. 151*		✔		dumbbells, bench
Dumbbell Shoulder Press, *p. 124*	✔			dumbbells, exercise ball
Slam Dunk, *p. 121*	✔			medicine ball
Triceps Push-down, *p. 127*	✔			cable machine
Tubing Kickback, *p. 125*	✔			tubing
Tubing Stroke, *p. 123*	✔			tubing

UPPER BACK (latissimus dorsi, trapezius, rhomboids)	SWIM	BIKE	RUN	EQUIPMENT
Barbell Row, *p. 181*			✔	barbell
Bridging Pullover, *p. 122*	✔			tubing, exercise ball

Continued

UPPER BACK (latissimus dorsi, trapezius, rhomboids) *Continued*	SWIM	BIKE	RUN	EQUIPMENT
Dumbbell Angled Raise, *p. 133*	✔			dumbbells
Dumbbell Lateral Raise, *p. 132*	✔			dumbbells
One-Arm Throw, *p. 120*	✔			tubing
Retraction, *p. 178*			✔	tubing
Shoulder Dip, *p. 154*		✔		dip stand
Slam Dunk, *p. 121*	✔			medicine ball
Tubing Row, *p. 179*			✔	tubing
Tubing Stroke, *p. 123*	✔			tubing
WRISTS/FOREARMS	SWIM	BIKE	RUN	EQUIPMENT
Barbell Wrist Curl, *p. 156*		✔		bench, barbell
Overhand Curl, *p. 159*		✔		barbell

LOWER-BODY EXERCISES

ANKLE/DORSIFLEXORS	SWIM	BIKE	RUN	EQUIPMENT
Cable Toe Raise, *p. 191*			✔	cable machine
Lying Hip Flex, *p. 165*		✔		cable machine
Seated Toe Raise, *p. 192*			✔	bench, plates
Toe Taps, *p. 170*		✔		bench
CALVES	SWIM	BIKE	RUN	EQUIPMENT
Leg Press, *p. 193*			✔	machine
One-Leg Squat, *p. 163*		✔		none (wall)
Seated Calf Raise, *p. 142*	✔			machine
Single-Calf Raise, *p. 167*		✔		step
Split Squat, *p. 185*			✔	dumbbells

CALVES *Continued*	SWIM	BIKE	RUN	EQUIPMENT
Squat, *p. 186*			✔	squat cage, bar, plates
Standing Calf Raise, *p. 143*	✔			step
Step-up, *p. 164*		✔		dumbbells, step
Walking Lunge, *p. 162*		✔		dumbbells
GLUTES	SWIM	BIKE	RUN	EQUIPMENT
Cable Hip Extension, *p. 139*	✔			cable machine
Cable Lateral Lift, *p. 136*	✔			cable machine
Dumbbell Deep Squat, *p. 171*		✔		dumbbells
Glute Lift, *p. 196*			✔	ankle weights, exercise ball
Inclined Superman, *p. 137*	✔			exercise ball
Lateral Lunge, *p. 145*	✔			dumbbells
Leg Press, *p. 193*			✔	machine
Lying Leg Lift, *p. 144*	✔			ankle weights
One-Leg Squat, *p. 163*		✔		none (wall)
Prone Extension, *p. 146*	✔			ankle weights
Reverse Lunge, *p. 172*		✔		dumbbells
Romanian Deadlift, *p. 194*			✔	barbell
Split Squat, *p. 185*			✔	dumbbells
Squat, *p. 186*			✔	squat cage, bar, plates
Step-up, *p. 164*		✔		dumbbells, step
Walking Lunge, *p. 162*		✔		dumbbells

Continued

HAMSTRINGS	SWIM	BIKE	RUN	EQUIPMENT
Cable Hip Extension, p. 139	✔			cable machine
Dumbbell Deep Squat, p. 171		✔		dumbbells
Glute Lift, p. 196			✔	ankle weights, exercise ball
Inclined Superman, p. 137	✔			exercise ball
Knee Raise, p. 166		✔		dip stand
Lateral Lunge, p. 145	✔			dumbbells
Leg Press, p. 193			✔	machine
Lying Hip Flex, p. 165		✔		cable machine
Lying Leg Curl, p. 141	✔			machine
Lying Single-Leg Curl, p. 190			✔	machine
Reverse Lunge, p. 172		✔		dumbbells
Romanian Deadlift, p. 194			✔	barbell
Seated Leg Curl, p. 169		✔		machine
Split Squat, p. 185			✔	dumbbells
Squat, p. 186			✔	squat cage, bar, plates
Standing Leg Curl, p. 189			✔	ankle weights
HIP FLEXORS/ADDUCTORS	SWIM	BIKE	RUN	EQUIPMENT
Cable Hip Flex, p. 188			✔	cable machine
Cable Lateral Cross, p. 140	✔			cable machine
Knee Raise, p. 166		✔		dip stand
Lying Hip Flex, p. 165		✔		cable machine
Medicine Ball Pike, p. 195			✔	medicine ball

QUADRICEPS	SWIM	BIKE	RUN	EQUIPMENT
Cable Hip Flex, *p. 188*			✔	cable machine
Dumbbell Deep Squat, *p. 171*		✔		dumbbells
Lateral Lunge, *p. 145*	✔			dumbbells
Leg Extension, *p. 138*	✔			machine
Leg Press, *p. 193*			✔	machine
One-Leg Squat, *p. 163*		✔		none (wall)
Reverse Lunge, *p. 172*		✔		dumbbells
Single-Leg Extension, *p. 168*		✔		machine
Split Squat, *p. 185*			✔	dumbbells
Squat, *p. 186*			✔	squat cage, bar, plates
Step-up, *p. 164*		✔		dumbbells, step
Walking Lunge, *p. 162*		✔		dumbbells

APPENDIX B

Muscular Endurance Exercises

What follows are body weight exercises and exercises that use smaller loads or resistance to build strength—ankle weights, medicine balls, or tubing. Because they require minimal equipment, these exercises are well suited for travel and home workouts.

		BODY-WEIGHT EXERCISES
EXERCISE	**REPS**	**OTHER EQUIPMENT**
Combination Crunch, *p. 105*	2 × 20	exercise ball
Inclined Superman, *p. 137*	3 × 15	exercise ball
Modified Sit-up, *p. 107*	2 × 10	—
Moguls, *p. 109*	2 × 20	exercise ball
One-Leg Squat, *p. 163*	2 × 10	—
Single-Calf Raise, *p. 167*	3 × 25	—
Stability Ball Bridge, *p. 108*	4 × 60 sec.	exercise ball
Standing Calf Raise, *p. 143*	3 × 20	—
Toe Taps, *p. 170*	3 × 60 sec.	—
V-up, *p. 106*	2 × 20	—

Continued

BODY-WEIGHT EXERCISES FOR THE GYM

EXERCISE	REPS	OTHER EQUIPMENT
Back Extension, *p. 149*	3 × 15	back extension bench
Dip, *p. 131*	3 × 10	dip stand
Dumbbell Handle Push-up, *p. 152*	3 × 20	dumbbells
Knee Raise, *p. 166*	3 × 25	dip stand
Shoulder Dip, *p. 154*	3 × 10	dip stand

ANKLE WEIGHT EXERCISES

EXERCISE	REPS	OTHER EQUIPMENT
Glute Lift, *p. 196*	2 × 10	medicine ball or dumbbells
Lying Leg Lift, *p. 144*	3 × 20	—
Prone Extension, *p. 146*	2 × 15	—
Standing Leg Curl, *p. 189*	3 × 15	—

MEDICINE BALL EXERCISES

EXERCISE	REPS	OTHER EQUIPMENT
Lunging Russian Twist, *p. 115*	2 × 30	—
Lying Russian Twist, *p. 116*	3 × 10	—
Medicine Ball Pike, *p. 195*	2 × 10	—
Pendulum, *p. 117*	3 × 20	—
Slam Dunk, *p.121*	2 × 15	—
Standing Russian Twist, *p. 114*	3 × 20	—
Stump Throw, *p. 113*	2 × 20	—

TUBING EXERCISES		
EXERCISE	**REPS**	**OTHER EQUIPMENT**
Bridging Pullover, *p. 122*	3 × 15	exercise ball
Diagonal Wood Chop, *p. 110*	2 × 20	—
One-Arm Throw, *p. 120*	2 × 15	—
Protraction, *p. 150*	3 × 15	—
Retraction, *p. 178*	3 × 15	—
Tubing Kickback, *p. 125*	2 × 15	—
Tubing Row, *p. 179*	3 × 15	—
Tubing Stroke, *p. 123*	3 × 15	—
Two-Arm Throw, *p. 112*	2–4 × 15	—

Exercise Log of Goal Weights Based on 1-Rep Max

For detailed instructions on how to determine your 1-rep max, refer back to Chapter 2 (pages 23–27). Remember that for more strenuous exercises you can estimate your 1-rep max from a submaximal lift using Table 2.3 (see p. 25).

EXERCISE	1RM	MUSCULAR ENDURANCE 50–67%	HYPER-TROPHY 65–85%	POWER/ STRENGTH 80–100%
Barbell Front Raise, *p. 157*				
Barbell Lift, *p. 180*				
Barbell Row, *p. 181*				
Barbell Wrist Curl, *p. 156*				
Bench Press, *p. 158*				
Cable Hip Extension, *p. 139*				
Cable Lateral Cross, *p. 140*				
Cable Lateral Lift, *p. 136*				
Dumbbell Angled Raise, *p. 133*				
Dumbbell Curl, *p. 126*				

Continued

EXERCISE	1RM	MUSCULAR ENDURANCE 50–67%	HYPER-TROPHY 65–85%	POWER/ STRENGTH 80–100%
Dumbbell Deep Squat, *p. 171*				
Dumbbell Fly, *p. 128*				
Dumbbell French Curl, *p. 182*				
Dumbbell Front Raise, *p. 155*				
Dumbbell Incline Press, *p. 151*				
Dumbbell Lateral Raise, *p. 132*				
Dumbbell Shoulder Press, *p. 124*				
Hammer Curl, *p. 174*				
Lateral Lunge, *p. 145*				
Leg Extension, *p. 138*				
Lying Hip Flex, *p. 165*				
Lying Leg Curl, *p. 141*				
Overhand Curl, *p. 159*				
Reverse Lunge, *p. 172*				
Runner's Raise, *p. 175*				
Seated Calf Raise, *p. 142*				
Seated Leg Curl, *p. 169*				
Shrug, *p. 177*				
Single-Leg Extension, *p. 168*				
Squat, *p. 186*				
Step-up, *p. 164*				
Triceps Push-down, *p. 127*				
Upright Row, *p. 176*				
Walking Lunge, *p. 162*				

Index

About the Author

Dr. Patrick Hagerman, EdD, FNSCA, CSCS, NSCA-CPT, has established himself as an authority on the topic of strength training through his experience as a professor of exercise and sports science, a coach, and a personal trainer. Starting as a collegiate strength and conditioning coach, Hagerman went on to coach for USA Weightlifting and USA Triathlon and to serve on the USA Triathlon Coaching Commission.

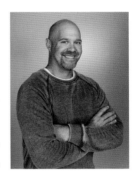

Hagerman is a fellow of the National Strength and Conditioning Association (NSCA), a past member of its board of directors, and a recipient of the 2002 NSCA Personal Trainer of the Year award.

Hagerman has written six other books on fitness and strength training, contributed to numerous textbooks, and published more than 30 articles on strength and conditioning.

For over 25 years he has competed in triathlon, cycling, windsurfing, and adventure racing, but in recent years his hobby of building custom hot rods has grown into a thriving business, Scotlea Hot Rods.

Hagerman lives in Bartlesville, Oklahoma, where he spends his free time coaching his kids' soccer, basketball, and baseball teams and collecting cars.

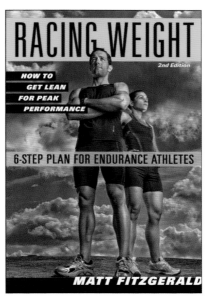
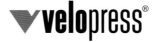